Contemporary Diagnosis and Management of

Obesity®

George A. Bray, MD

Professor,
Pennington Biomedical Research Center,
Louisiana State University,
Baton Rouge, Louisiana

Published by Handbooks in Health Care Co.,
Newtown, Pennsylvania, USA

International Standard Book Number: 1-884065-30-9

Library of Congress Catalog Card Number: 98-70972

Table of Contents

Appendices

Introduction

"Corpulency, when in an extraordinary degree, may be reckoned a disease, as it in some measure obstructs the free exercise of the animal functions; and hath a tendency to shorten life, by paving the way to dangerous distempers."

— Malcolm Flemyng (1760)

Obesity is a worldwide epidemic. Data from around the world show a steady increase in overweight since World War II. The epidemic has exploded in the past 10 years. In the United States, the percentage of people who are overweight has increased more than 30% since 1980. Similar sharp increases in the prevalence of obesity have occurred worldwide.

Many factors influence the development of obesity (Figure 1). At the center is the balance between the fat, carbohydrate, and protein food energy that people eat, and the energy they consume in daily living. Each of these is influenced by a variety of individual factors reflecting genes and metabolism, which are in turn modified by environmental and societal factors. The epidemic of overweight, however, must largely be environmental. I call it the *mismatch model*. There is a mismatch between the food energy people eat and what they need. The abundance of food and sedentary lifestyle are a mismatch for the ancient genetic makeup of most people who adapted when scarcity was the rule, surfeit a rarity. In some ethnic groups, almost everyone is overweight. Whether all ethnic groups will show this high prevalence in time, or whether significant genes for thinness exist, is not yet known.

The argument that the epidemic of overweight is largely environmental is important because it helps direct strate-

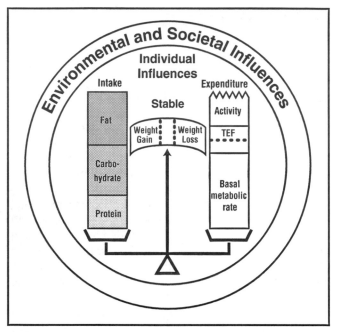

Figure 1: *Influences on the development of obesity.*

gies for prevention and treatment. Studies of ethnic groups that migrated from one dietary environment to another provide one source of data. Japanese who migrated to Hawaii and California are more overweight than relatives remaining in Japan. A similar fate awaited Chinese and African immigrants to Western culture.

Other data supporting important environmental factors come from studies of temporal changes within a country. In both China and Japan, increasing fat consumption paralleled the rise in the prevalence of overweight. In the United States, the increasing time spent in front of the television parallels the increase in overweight in children.

The rise in the percentage of dietary fat in the food supply of developing countries appears to be a factor in the increasing prevalence of overweight. Higher-fat diets have more calorically dense foods, and smaller amounts or weights of food are needed to provide for energy needs. Two strategies can address this problem. The first is to eat a lower-fat diet, directly decreasing energy density of the diet. The alternate strategy is to reduce the energy density of foods by other techniques. This second strategy can be applied where much food is processed. In developing countries, a different strategy may be needed that focuses on quantity of fat.

An increase in sedentary lifestyle is the other key element in the development of obesity. This must be reversed to prevent overweight from becoming preclinical or clinical overweight. Two approaches may be helpful. The first is to reduce the amount of time of inactivity. The second is to increase the amount of daily physical activity. These concepts of prevention and treatment are developed in the following chapters.

The preparation of this book depended on the invaluable input of many people. The continuing intellectual stimulation by my current and former fellows and colleagues, particularly Dr. David York, Dr. Donna Ryan, and Dr. Frank Greenway, is gratefully acknowledged. The support of my wife was essential for timely completion. The preparation of the text is the work of Ms. Terry Hodges, Ms. Cheryl Shuffield, and Ms. Janice Warren. Ms. Hodges also did many of the illustrations. I am indebted to all of them.

Dedication

To my wife and children,
for their forbearance and tolerance.

Chapter 1

Who are the Obese? Body Composition and Prevalence

"Measure what can be measured, and make measurable what cannot be measured."

— Galileo Galilei

Obesity is common in the United States and elsewhere. The increasing number of overweight Americans is accompanied by increased health risks and increased demands on the health-care system for advice and treatment. We need a set of ground rules that define overweight and obesity. The definitions are simple, but the way they are applied is more complex.

Definitions

Obesity is any increase in body fat. In its extreme, it can be easily diagnosed visually. This increase in fat can be evenly distributed over the body, or it can be concentrated in specific regions. Differences in body fat distribution are particularly obvious between men and women. Increased amounts of fat in females soften contours and reduce angularity of muscles and joints. In men, however, the smaller quantity of fat for any given weight and size makes muscles, bones, and joints appear more angular. Women tend to deposit fat more on their buttocks and thighs, and men tend to deposit it on their waist. These gender differences in fat deposition have led to descriptions of android or upper-body obesity for the

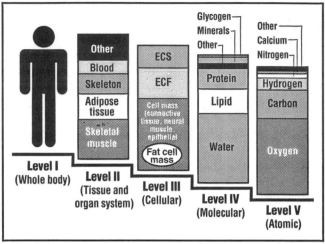

Figure 1: Five perspectives on body composition. The human body is classified into increasingly general categories, from the atomic level through the molecular, cellular, tissue-system, and whole-body levels. Each perspective is characterized by a set of unique components that define its measurement parameters.[5]

'male' type, and gynoid or lower-body fat distribution for the 'female' pattern. However, these patterns occur in both genders.

Overweight is an increase in weight relative to some standard. The nature of that standard is addressed in Chapter 5 with the development of criteria for the tools to evaluate overweight.

Methods for determining body composition have improved over the past 25 years, greatly increasing the accuracy and ease of measuring body compartments in patients.[1-4] Body composition measurements may be useful in making clinical judgments for nutritional therapy in undernourished patients. Measures such as body mass index (BMI) and waist circumference are the minimum clinical criteria for evaluating overweight patients. Body composition also may be useful in identifying patients in whom total body fat may not be much increased but visceral fat is significantly increased, a setting that substantially increases the risk of heart disease and diabetes. This chapter reviews body composition and methods of measurement.

Body Composition

The human body can be analyzed from many perspectives. A 5-level model is shown in Figure 1.[5] These five levels reflect improvements over the past 5 centuries in the methods of examining the human body. The initial studies of the human body during the Renaissance were done for artistic purposes, which required studies of the underlying anatomic structure. Vesalius published the first modern anatomy of the human body in 1543. With the invention of the microscope in the 17th century, the tissue (Level II) and cellular levels (Level III) of the human body were gradually unveiled. This was followed in the 19th and 20th centuries by improvements in chemistry and physics that allowed for a molecular (Level IV) and atomic (Level V) understanding of body composition. A similar progression occurred in pathology: organ pathology preceded tissue pathology, which in turn preceded cellular and molecular pathology.

Whole Body (Level I)

The first level of analysis of body composition is the whole body (Level I). Wang et al identified at least 10 different measurable components, including stature (height), length of limbs, various circumferences including waist and hips, skinfold thickness at various sites (eg, triceps, subscapular), body surface area, body volume, BMI, and body density.[5] The measurement of BMI and the circumference of the waist and hips are emphasized in the section marked **Overweight**.

Tissue and Organ Composition (Level II)

The division of the body into organs and tissues is obvious. Five major tissues are shown in Figure 1, including skeletal muscle, adipose tissue, skeleton, blood or hematopoietic tissues, and all others. The amount and location of adipose tissue are most important. As much as 80% of body fat is subcutaneous; however, fat also surrounds many organs and accumulates around the abdominal organs. Fat in this latter category is most difficult to measure accurately except with expensive imaging techniques.

Cellular Composition (Level III)

A third level in the analysis of body composition is the cellular components. The body is composed of cells in all tissues and organs, which have intracellular fluid and are surrounded by extracellular fluids and solids. Figure 1 lists two major cellular categories. These include connective-tissue cells, neural cells, muscle cells, epithelial cells, and the fat cells that we are most concerned about in obesity. One technique for measuring body cell mass uses the naturally occurring radioactive isotope of potassium (^{40}K). Because more than 95% of potassium is intracellular, the ability to measure an isotope of potassium provides an index of body cell mass. ^{40}K is a naturally occurring isotope of potassium, and its abundance can be determined with whole-body radiation counters. Total body weight is the sum of all tissues, including muscle cells, connective-tissue cells, epithelial cells, and neural cells. The metabolically active tissues, such as bone, adipose tissue, blood cells, and muscle, make up 75% of body weight.

Molecular Composition (Level IV)

This part of the model is most widely used in clinical medicine. Water constitutes 60% or more of the weight in males, and 50% in females. Of this 60%, approximately 26% is extracellular and 34% intracellular. Lipids range

Table 1: Criteria for Obesity in Males and Females

Category	Body Fat Males	Females
Normal	12%-20%	20%-30%
Borderline	21%-25%	31%-33%
Obesity	>25%	>33%

from less than 10% of body weight in well-trained athletes to nearly 50% in obese patients. Two percent to 3% of these lipids are essential structural lipids, and the remainder are nonessential stores. Protein constitutes 15% of normal body composition, and minerals constitute 5.3%. Thus, water, lipid, protein, and minerals account for 99.4% of the molecular constituents of the body.

Several molecular models can be used to describe body weight. The most widely used clinical model comprises two compartments: the sum of fat and the fat-free mass.

1. Body weight = fat + fat-free mass (FFM)

More complex models can be developed by subdividing fat-free mass into other molecular components. One 4-compartment model is:

2. Body weight = fat + water + protein + bone mineral

The model obtained from dual energy x-ray absorptiometry (see below) has three compartments:

3. Body weight = fat + bone mineral + lean body mass

The amount of fat in the body varies more widely than any other single component. Table 1 provides a range of body fat values for normal, borderline, and obese men and women.

Data from dissection studies and from all indirect measures clearly show that women have a higher percentage

Table 2: Methods for Measuring Body Composition

	Cost
Anthropometry	
Height and weight	$
Diameters	$
Circumferences	$
Skinfolds	$
Instrumental	
Hydrodensitometry	$$
Air displacement • plethysmography	$$$$
Dual x-ray absorptiometry (DXA)	$$$
Isotope dilution	$$
Impedance (BIA)	$$
^{40}K counting	$$$$
Conductivity (TOBEC)	$$$
CT	$$$$
MRI	$$$$
Neutron activation	$$$$
Ultrasound	$$

*Special equipment; $=inexpensive; $$=more expensive; $$$=expensive; $$$$=very expensive; E=easy; M=moderately difficult; D=difficult

of body fat than do men. Values of well below 10% fat have been reported in highly trained long-distance runners, but as the values get lower, the precision of the measurement worsens and the reliability of these numbers is sometimes questionable. At the other extreme, body fat

Ease of use	Can measure regional fat	External radiation
E	no	
E	+	
E	+	
M	+	
E*	no	
D*	no	
M*	+	trace
M*	no	
E*	+	
D*	no	
D*	±	
D*	++	some
D*	++	
D*	no	larger
M*	+	

+ = good
++ = very good
± = possibly

can rise to more than 50% of total body weight, but rarely above 60%. The very large majority of this fat is stored in droplets in the 40 billion to 60 billion adipocytes in the adult human body. A small quantity of lipid is associated with membrane structures and is considered essential.

Proteins provide the structural and functional components of the body. Approximately 15% of the body is protein, but this varies with age and degree of physical training, and with a variety of clinical and hormonal states. Many minerals constitute the remainder of the body's molecular structure. Water, lipid, protein, and mineral account for more than 99% of the molecular constituents of the body.

Atomic Composition (Level V)

A final model of the human body partitions it into atomic components. If the standard or reference man is 70 kg, this individual's weight would be 60% oxygen, 23% carbon, 10% hydrogen, 2.6% nitrogen, 1.4% calcium, and less than 1% assigned to all of the other atoms in the body, such as chloride, copper, fluoride, chromium, magnesium, potassium, phosphorus, sodium, sulfur, nickel, zinc, and others. Eleven elements thus account for more than 99.5% of body weight. Oxygen, carbon, hydrogen, nitrogen, and calcium account for more than 98% of total body mass. Less than 2% is attributable to the other atomic elements. The other atomic components of clinical interest are nitrogen, calcium, magnesium, sodium, potassium, and chloride.[5]

Several methods have been proposed for measuring body fat and fat distribution. These run from simple and inexpensive techniques to complex and very expensive. Table 2 groups these methods in 2 categories: anthropometric and instrumental.

Anthropometric Measures

For the first group of measurements, a tape measure, balance scale, and skinfold caliper are the only needed instruments. This is not true for the instrumental methods; thus, their costs often are much higher. The standard manual by Lohman et al provides detailed descriptions of how to use these methods.[6] The following leans heavily on this expert manual. Accurate measurement of height and weight is essential in the clinical evaluation of all patients (Chapter 5). Height and weight should be determined by calibrated stadiometer and scales. BMI can be calculated from height and weight. Waist circumference, and sometimes hip circumference are measured. Determining skinfold thickness for clinical purposes is not recommended.

The accuracy and reliability of the measurements are greatest for height and weight. Circumferences and diameters are next, and skinfolds are a distant third. An additional problem with skinfolds is that, in overweight patients, some skinfolds may be too thick to be measured with calipers. Therefore, skinfolds are not widely used clinically.

Instrumental Methods

The number and precision of methods for measuring body composition has improved greatly over the past 25 years. These allow for measurement of most body compartments with as much precision as needed, if cost is no issue (Table 2).

Dual X-Ray Absorptiometry (DXA)

DXA instruments were developed for determination of bone mineral content as part of an evaluation of osteoporosis. The method requires the subject to lie supine on a table. Two very low-energy x-ray beams of different energy are passed through the body. The x-ray beams are attenuated to estimate lean body mass, body fat, and bone mineral content.[2] DXA has replaced underwater weighing in many laboratories as the gold standard for determining body fat and lean body mass. The advantages of DXA are:

- It can be safely applied to all ranges of individuals up to 150 kg (300 lb).
- It is easy to use.
- With appropriate standards, it is very accurate.

The disadvantages of DXA are:
- High cost of the instrument, between $40,000 and $100,000
- The need for regular cross-standardization of the instrument
- The weight limits of the table, which prevent measurement for individuals weighing more than 150 kg

The reproducibility of DXA is 0.8% for bone, 1.3% for density, 1.7% for fat, and 2.0% for body weight. The radiation exposure with this procedure is barely higher than normal background radiation, and well below that of a chest x-ray.

Hydrodensitometry

Determining body density and partitioning it into fat and nonfat compartments, based on the fact that fat floats and the nonfat components sink, was the gold standard of body composition until the advent of DXA.[2] Its advantages are that it is highly reproducible, easy to perform, and requires only a good balance. Its disadvantage is that some individuals are unable or unwilling to completely submerge in water. Measurement of pulmonary residual volume at the time of the test is an important secondary method required to increase the accuracy of this procedure. Air displacement is similar in principle, but does not require submersion.

Bioelectric Impedance Analysis (BIA)

Measurement of the resistance and impedance of the body between predetermined points on the leg and arm or between feet and arms has been widely used to determine water content.[1] With proper training and careful placement of electrodes, highly reproducible measurements can be obtained. The instrument for this procedure costs between $2,000 and $3,000, and is portable. The advantages of this method are its relatively low cost and its ease of performance from the subject's point of view, and the ability to compare with other centers that use similar instrumentation. The disadvantages include that the impedance only adds a small amount of extra information to the other pieces of information, such as height and age, required for the equations. Second, the method is indirect because it only measures body water, which is used to estimate body fat. Several precautions are needed to obtain valid information from BIA. First, the instrumentation must be reliable. Second, the procedures must be standardized by using the same time of the day, the same ambient temperature, and standard placement of electrodes. Third, the subject should be similar to the populations from which the standard values are derived. Finally, the subject's water status should be stable because BIA measures water.

Infrared Reactance

This technique involves the application of an infrared signal over the biceps, where reflectance is read and acts as a signal for underlying fatness. No commercially acceptable unit yet embodies this technology, and it is not clinically recommended.

Total Body Electrical Conductivity

Two instruments, one for adults and one for children, have been developed that use total body conductivity (TOBEC). The principle is similar to the methods of evaluating fat content of meat through changes in electromagnetic fields that depend on the relation of fat and water. Like DXA, the TOBEC instrument is expensive, but it may be useful in a research setting, particularly for children.[2]

Imaging Techniques

Regional body fat distribution can be reliably determined by either computed tomography (CT) or magnetic

Table 3:	Techniques for Evaluating Body Weight

- Life insurance tables
- Relative weight $= \dfrac{\text{actual weight}}{\text{desirable weight}} \times 100$
- Body mass index (kg/m²)

resonance imaging (MRI).[4,7] CT uses x-radiation and computer analysis to determine the structure of internal organs. An accuracy of less than 1% error for body fat is possible with a series of scans. To minimize radiation dose, however, a single cut at the L4-L5 position is used for measurement of visceral and subcutaneous fat. MRI requires a powerful magnet that surrounds the subject. It has no risks, but takes longer to perform than CT. Because movement blurs the images, MRI cannot evaluate the heart. The estimates of subcutaneous and visceral fat obtained by these two methods may differ in absolute terms, but the relative ranking among subjects is similar.

Careful measurement of height, weight, and waist circumference are the minimal measurements needed to begin evaluation of an overweight patient (Chapter 5). If the clinician is concerned about whether fat is increased, DXA may be beneficial. Although impedance measurements are used in many clinical settings, they do not contribute more than do the methods outlined above. Expensive techniques, such as whole-body potassium count and neutron activation analysis, obtain information about body cell mass using naturally occurring potassium or the calcium and nitrogen content from neutron activation. This technology is limited in availability, is extremely expensive, and produces significant radiation.

Table 4: Classification of Overweight and Obesity in Adults According to BMI

Classification	BMI (kg/m^2)*	Risk of comorbidities**
Underweight	<18.5	Low (but risk of other clinical problems increased)
Normal range	18.5-24.9	Average
Overweight	25.0-29.9	Mildly increased
Obese	≥30.0	
Class I	30.0-34.9	Moderate
Class II	35.0-39.9	Severe
Class III	≥40.0	Very severe

*Values are age independent and the same for both sexes. However, BMI may not correspond to the same degree of fatness across different populations.

**Both BMI and a measure of fat distribution (eg, waist circumference, waist/hip ratio) are important in calculating the risk of obesity comorbidities. BMI <18.5 kg/m^2 signifies an increased risk of developing other clinical problems.

Adapted from WHO[21] and the National Heart, Lung, and Blood Institute: *Clinical Guidelines on the Identification, Evaluation, and Treatment of Overweight and Obesity in Adults*, June 1998.

Regional Fat

Table 2 lists methods that can be used for estimating the distribution of body fat. Skinfolds and, alternatively, ultrasound can estimate subcutaneous fat thickness. Measurement at several sites can assess regional fat localization, but these techniques do not help in assessing visceral fat. The gold standard for measuring visceral fat is CT or MRI scan of a cross-section of the abdomen (see above).

Table 5: A Table of Body Mass Index (BMI)

	Good Weights									
Height	19	20	21	22	23	24	25	26	27	28
4'10"	91	96	100	105	110	115	119	124	129	134
4'11"	94	99	104	109	114	119	124	128	133	138
5'	97	102	107	112	118	123	128	133	138	143
5'1"	100	106	111	116	122	127	132	137	143	148
5'2"	104	109	115	120	126	131	136	142	147	153
5'3"	107	113	118	124	130	135	141	146	152	158
5'4"	110	116	122	128	134	140	145	151	157	163
5'5"	114	120	126	132	138	144	150	156	162	168
5'6"	118	124	130	136	142	148	155	161	167	173
5'7"	121	127	134	140	146	153	159	166	172	178
5'8"	125	131	138	144	151	158	164	171	177	184
5'9"	128	135	142	149	155	162	169	176	182	189
5'10"	132	139	146	153	160	167	174	181	188	195
5'11"	136	143	150	157	165	172	179	186	193	200
6'	140	147	154	162	169	177	184	191	199	206
6'1"	144	151	159	166	174	182	189	197	204	212
6'2"	148	155	163	171	179	186	194	202	210	218
6'3"	152	160	168	176	184	192	200	208	216	224
6'4"	156	164	172	180	189	197	205	213	221	230

					Increasing Risk						
29	**30**	**31**	**32**	**33**	**34**	**35**	**36**	**37**	**38**	**39**	**40**
138	143	148	153	158	162	167	172	177	181	186	191
143	148	153	158	163	168	173	178	183	188	193	198
148	153	158	163	168	174	179	184	189	194	199	204
153	158	164	169	174	180	185	190	195	201	206	211
158	164	169	175	180	186	191	196	202	207	213	218
163	169	175	180	186	191	197	203	208	214	220	225
169	174	180	186	192	197	204	209	215	221	227	232
174	180	186	192	198	204	210	216	222	228	234	240
179	186	192	198	204	210	216	223	229	235	241	247
185	191	198	204	211	217	223	230	236	242	249	255
190	197	203	210	216	223	230	236	243	249	256	262
196	203	209	216	223	230	236	243	250	257	263	270
202	209	216	222	229	236	243	250	257	264	271	278
208	215	222	229	236	243	250	257	265	272	279	286
213	221	228	235	242	250	258	265	272	279	287	294
219	227	235	242	250	257	265	272	280	288	295	302
225	233	241	249	256	264	272	280	287	295	303	311
232	240	248	256	264	272	279	287	295	303	311	319
238	246	254	263	271	279	287	295	304	312	320	328

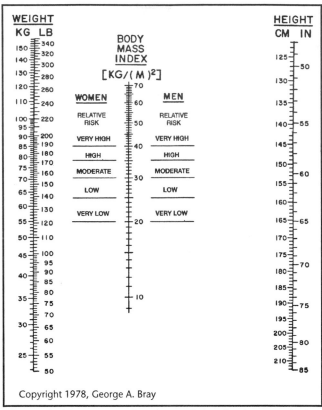

Figure 2: Nomogram for determining body mass index. Place a ruler or other straight edge between the body weight in kilograms or pounds (without clothes) on the left-hand line, and the height in centimeters or in inches (without shoes) on the right-hand line. The body mass index is read from the middle of the scale in metric units (copyright 1978, George A. Bray. Used with permission).

Three measurements have received the most evaluation: (1) circumference of the waist divided by the circumference of the hips (WHR). This procedure was used in several seminal studies showing the importance of central fat distribution in the risk of disease (Chapter 4); (2) sagittal diameter measured as the diameter from the abdomen to the back; (3) waist circumference alone. In comparative studies, waist circumference alone is as good as either WHR or sagittal diameter. Therefore, measurement of height and weight, measurement of waist circumference, and, when available, measurement of bioelectric impedance or DXA are the standard tools for assessing the impact of body fat on health risk (see Chapter 3).

Overweight

Overweight is an increase in body weight relative to some standard. Table 3 lists three techniques for evaluating degree of overweight. The first is the life insurance table, or the ratio of actual weight divided by the 'desirable' weight. Relative weight is the weight of an individual compared to a table, usually the Metropolitan Life Insurance Table. BMI is the third and most widely used standard for determining overweight. BMI is body weight in kilograms divided by the square of stature in meters (kg/m^2), and was originally proposed by Quetelet more than 150 years ago. It correlates more closely with body fat content than do other anthropometric relationships of height and weight, and thus is the preferred measure in epidemiologic and population studies. Its advantages are ease of determination and the accuracy in measuring both height (stature) and weight. Its chief limitation is that, particularly in the normal BMI range (18.5-24.9 kg/m^2), the correlation with actual body fat content is sufficiently low that it is a poor guide to individual fat level. For BMI values above 25 kg/m^2 and especially above 30 kg/m^2, it is a much better guide to the degrees of excess fat and risk to health.

Table 4 lists BMI ranges and the relative risk associated with each. This concept of BMI and risk is explored in more detail in chapters 3 and 5, which outline the clini-

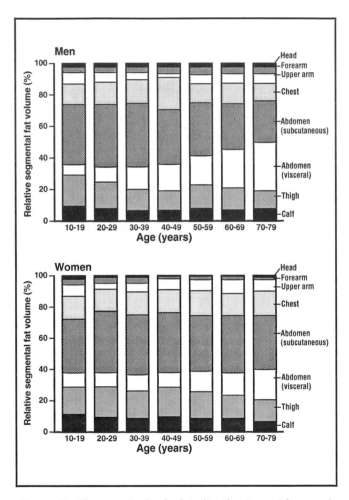

Figure 3: *Changes in body fat distribution with age. In men, shown at the top, the percentage of abdominal or visceral fat steadily increases with age, and fat in the calf and in the abdominal subcutaneous area decreases. In women, the rise in abdominal or visceral fat largely occurs after the menopause.*[9]

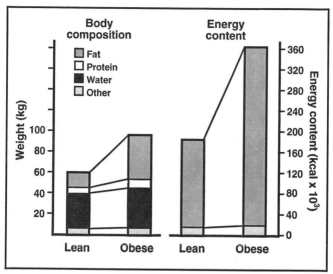

Figure 4: *Body composition in lean and obese individuals who differ by 30 kg. The measured components are on the left, and the calculated energy content on the left shows that most of the energy is stored in fat. Energy content nearly doubles with a 50% increase in body weight.*

cal evaluation of overweight patients. A table and nomogram for estimating BMI are shown in Table 5 and Figure 2.[8] This index is in metric terms (kg/m^2). Calculating BMI using pounds and inches provides numbers that are very different from those in the table or the nomogram. The normal range of BMI is 18.5 to 25 kg/m^2.

Body Composition Through the Life Span

Several factors modify the level of body fat and body composition, including gender, age, level of physical activity, and hormonal status. Figure 3 shows the data on body fat distribution by age for men and women.[9] Two important observations are evident from this figure. First,

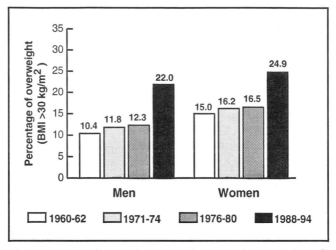

Figure 5: Prevalence of overweight (BMI above 30 kg/m²) in four surveys. Note the sudden jump in the percentage of overweight individuals in the most recent survey.[10]

percentage of body fat steadily increases with age in both men and women. Women have a higher percentage of body fat than do men for a comparable height and weight at any age. Second, visceral fat in women is lower during the reproductive years, but rises rapidly to nearly male levels in the postmenopausal years, when risk for cardiovascular and other diseases increases sharply. Indeed, corrections for differences in body fat distribution correct for almost all of the differences in excess mortality of men over women, suggesting that the underlying factors leading to differences in fat distribution are significant in the risk of diabetes, heart disease, high blood pressure, and stroke in men.

Body Composition and Obesity

Using some of the methods described earlier, we can compare body composition and its energetic equivalent

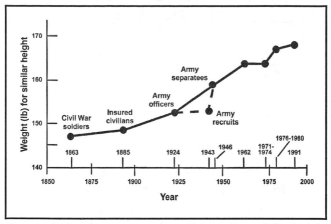

Figure 6: *Secular increase in weight adjusted for height over the past 150 years.*[20]

in men and women of two different weights. This is presented in Figure 4, which shows the effect of a 30-kg increase in weight for the standard 70-kg man and the standard 56-kg woman. More than two thirds of this increase in weight in men, and up to 90% in women, is accounted for by increased fat. The remainder is lean tissue that supports the extra fat. Because the extra stored triglyceride is energy rich, the 30-kg increase in weight nearly doubles body energy stores. The therapeutic challenge for treating obesity thus is to reduce this excess energy stored in body fat without disproportionate loss in lean tissue associated with fat storage.

Prevalence of Overweight

Using BMI, we can divide the population into groups and compare these groups across national boundaries, and examine time trends. The mean BMI for women is slightly lower than for men (26.6 kg/m² for men, 26.5 kg/m² for women). The median BMI is 25.9 kg/m² for men and

29

Table 6: Trends in Obesity (BMI ≥ 30 kg/m^2) by Country

Population	Year	Age	Prevalence of Obesity (%)	
			Men	Women
USA[10]	1960	20-74	10.4	15.0
	1971-74		11.8	16.2
	1976-80		12.3	16.5
	1988-1991		20.0	24.9
Canada	1978[11]	20-70	6.8	9.6
	1981[12]	20-70	8.5	9.3
	1998[13]	20-70	9.0	9.2
	1986-92[a]	18-74	13.0	14.0
Brazil[14]	1975	25-64	3.1	8.2
	1989		5.9	13.3
England[15]	1980	16-64	6.0	8.0
	1986-87		7	12
	1991		12.7	15.0
	1994[b]		13.2	16.0
	1995[c]		15.0	16.5
Finland[16]	1978-79	20-75	10	10
	1985-87		12	10
	1991-93		14	11

25.1 kg/m^2 for women, resulting in greater skew, that is, the long upper tail is greater for women, giving them a higher percentage with a BMI above 30 kg/m^2 than for men.

The percentage of Americans with a BMI above 25 kg/m^2 or 30 kg/m^2 has been determined in several surveys by the American government, beginning in 1960.[10] These

Population	Year	Age	Prevalence of Obesity (%)	
			Men	Women
Netherlands[17]	1987	20-59	6.0	8.5
	1988		6.3	7.6
	1989		6.2	7.4
	1990		7.4	9.0
	1991		7.5	8.8
	1992		7.5	9.3
	1993		7.1	9.1
	1994		8.8	9.4
	1995		8.4	8.3
Japan[18]	1976	20+	0.7	2.8
	1982		0.9	2.6
	1987		1.3	2.8
	1993		1.8	2.6
China[19]	1989	20-45	0.29	0.89
	1991		0.36	0.86

[a] Reeder et al, 1992
[b] Colhoun H et al, 1996
[c] Prescott-Clarke P et al, 1997

data are plotted in Figure 5. The percentage of men and women exceeding a BMI of 30 kg/m^2 steadily increased in each of the first three surveys. There was a striking rise between the 3rd and 4th survey. The increase in percentage of men with a BMI above 30 kg/m^2 nearly doubled, and the percentage of women with a BMI above 30 kg/m^2

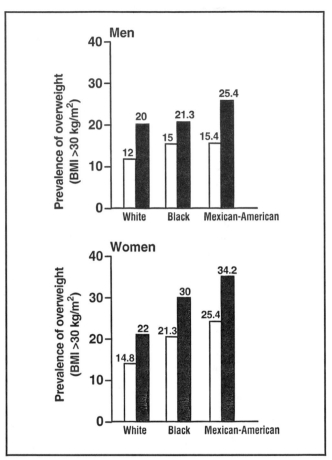

Figure 7: *Obesity in three ethnic groups using data from two different surveys by the National Center for Health Statistics.*[10]

rose by more than 50%. The rise in body weight relative to height is not new.[20] Figure 6 shows the rise in weight since the Civil War for men of the same height. What is new is the rate of this rise.

The epidemic of overweight is not confined to the United States, but can be identified in data from all over the world.[21] The data from several countries are shown in Table 6. The prevalence of overweight clearly is increasing worldwide in the Eastern and Western hemispheres, and above and below the equator. Despite the wide range, all data suggest that most populations have an increased percentage of overweight over the past 20 years.

The distribution of increased weight is not equally divided among the population.[10] Figure 7 shows the percentages of whites, blacks, and Mexican Americans in the United States with a BMI above 30 kg/m^2. Both Mexican Americans, and black women in particular, have high percentages of BMI above 30 kg/m^2.

The following chapters provide a background for understanding, prevention, and treatment of this epidemic.

References

1.   Bioelectrical Impedance Analysis in Body Composition Measurement. Proceedings of a National Institutes of Health Technology Assessment Conference. Bethesda, Maryland, December 12-14, 1994. *Am J Clin Nutr* 1996;64:387S-532S.

2.   Heymsfield SB, Allison DB, Wang ZM: Evaluation of total and regional body composition. In: Bray GA, Bouchard C, James WP, eds. *Handbook of Obesity.* New York, Marcel Dekker, 1997, pp 41-77.

3.   Lohman TG: *Advances in Body Composition Assessment.* Champaign, IL, Human Kinetics, 1992.

4.   Seidell JC, Rissanen AM: Time trends in worldwide prevalence of obesity. In: Bray GA, Bouchard C, James WP, eds. *Handbook of Obesity.* New York, Marcel Dekker, 1997, pp 79-91.

5.   Wang ZM, Pierson RN Jr, Heymsfield SB: The five-level model: a new approach to organizing body-composition research. *Am J Clin Nutr* 1992;56:19-28.

6.   Lohman TG, Roche AF, Martorell R: *Anthropometric Standardization Reference Manual.* Champaign, IL, Human Kinetics, 1988.

7.   Sjostrom L, Kvist H, Cederblad A, et al: Determination of total adipose tissue and body fat in women by computed tomography, ^{40}K, and tritium. *Am J Physiol* 1986;250:E736-E745.

8.   Bray GA, Gray DS: Obesity. Part I—Pathogenesis. *West J Med* 1988;149:429-441.

9.   Kotani KK, Tokunaga K, Fujioka S, et al: Sexual dimorphism of age-related changes in whole-body fat distribution in the obese. *Int J Obes Relat Metab Disord* 1994;18:207-212.

10. Flegal KM, Carroll MD, Kuczmarski RJ, et al: Overweight and obesity in the United States: prevalence and trends. *Int J Obes* 1998;22:39-47.

11. Health and Welfare Canada: *The Health of Canadians.* Report of the Canada Health Survey. Ottawa, Minister of Supplies and Services, Government of Canada, 1981.

12. *Canadian Standardized Test of Fitness: Operations Manual*, 3rd ed. Ottawa, Fitness Canada, 1986.

13. Stephens T, Craig CL: *The Well-Being of Canadians: Highlights of the 1988 Campbell's Survey.* Ottawa, Canadian Fitness and Lifestyle Research Institute, 1990.

14. Monteiro CA, Mondini L, de Souza AL, et al: The nutrition transition in Brazil. *Eur J Clin Nutr* 1995;49:105-113.

15. Kuskowska-Wolk A, Bergstrom R: Trends in body mass index and prevalence of obesity in Swedish women 1980-89. *J Epidemiol Community Health* 1993;47:195-199.

16. Seidell JS, Rissanen AM: Time trends in the worldwide prevalence of obesity. In: Bray GA, Bouchard C, James WP, eds. *Handbook of Obesity.* New York, Marcel Dekker, 1998, pp 79-91.

17. Seidell JC: Time trends in obesity: an epidemiological perspective. *Horm Metab Res* 1997;29:155-158.

18. Inoue S: Personal communication, based on interim data from the National Nutrition Survey in Japan from 1976 to 1993.

19. Chunming C: Personal communication, based on data from the 1992 China Nationwide Nutrition Survey.

20. Bray GA: The obese patient. In: *Major Problems in Internal Medicine, Vol. 9.* Philadelphia, WB Saunders, 1976, pp 1-450.

21. World Health Organization: *Obesity: Preventing and Managing the Global Epidemic.* Report of a WHO Consultation on Obesity, Geneva, June 1997.

Chapter 2

What Causes Overweight? Nature Versus Nurture

"Next to nature, there is nothing more wonderful than man's gradual understanding of it."
— George Sarton

*Talking to a man who had grown very fat
so as to be much incommoded by corpulency,
he said "He eats too much, Sir"
Boswell: I don't know, Sir. You will see one
man who eats moderately and another lean
who eats a great deal.
Johnson: Nay, Sir, whatever may be the quantity
that a man eats, it is plain that if he is too fat,
he has eaten more than he should have done.*
— Boswell's Life of Johnson

Obesity is a multifactorial disease. Each cause has a variable genetic component. At one extreme are the kinds of obesity that result from single-gene mutations, which usually produce massive obesity.[1,2] At the other extreme are the types of obesity produced by various experimental maneuvers or diseases in a setting where obesity would otherwise not occur. Damage to the ventromedial hypothalamus (VMH) of the brain is an example. This chapter first examines the obesities produced by single-gene defects. This is followed by a review of the genetic susceptibility that underlies human

Table 1: Single-Gene Animal Models of Obesity

Animal Model	Chromosome Rodent	Human Homolog	Gene Defect
Dominant Inheritance			
Yellow Mouse A^y (gene = Agouti)	2	20q 11.2	Agouti-signaling protein (ASP) overexpressed in many tissues
Recessive Inheritance			
Obese mouse (ob/ob) (gene = Lep)	6	7q 31.3	Stop codon 105 produces truncated leptin
Diabetes mouse (db/db)	4	1p 32	Splicing defects
Fatty rat (fa/fa) Koletsky rat fa^k/fa^k (gene = Lepr)	5		or extra-cellular deletions
Tub mouse (gene = tub)	7	4q 32	Insert
Fat mouse (gene = cpe)	8	11p 15	Insert

obesity. Finally, this chapter examines the physiologic and pathogenetic mechanisms that operate in this genetic framework to control food intake and energy expenditure, and to produce differences in total body fat and in regional fat distribution.

Gene Product	Reproductive Status	Mechanism
Asp (133 AA)	Slightly impaired	Competes with MSH for melanocortin receptors
Leptin (167 AA)	Infertile	Leptin signal from fat to brain and other organs
Leptin receptor (505 AA)	Infertile	Impaired leptin receptor
Phospho-diesterase (?)	Impaired	Hypothalamic; possible neuronal damage (apoptosis)
Carboxy-peptidase E	Impaired	Prohormones not cleaved

Genetic Models of Obesity
Animal Models

Table 1 summarizes the five single-gene defects that produce obesity in rodents. The first of these defects identified at the molecular level was the defect in the agouti gene, which produces the yellow obese mouse.[3] The agouti protein competes for the melanocortin receptor, a receptor system that may also be involved in human obesity. This agouti-signaling peptide is a 133-amino acid peptide that competes with melanocyte-stimulating hormone (MSH) at the melanocortin receptors in skin to prevent the formation of melanin, thus leading to a yellow mouse. The agouti-signaling protein also competes with α-MSH for a melanocortin receptor in the hypothalamus, which modulates food intake. Thus, the agouti-signaling protein can produce both the yellow coat color and the hyperphagia and obesity in this animal.

The ob or leptin gene in the obese mouse codes for a protein called leptin. This was the second defect described. Cloning of this gene by Zhang et al in 1994 was a major breakthrough in understanding one form of experimental obesity that has since been identified in humans.[4,5] Leptin-deficient mice are hyperphagic, hyperinsulinemic, insulin resistant, and infertile. Leptin administration reverses all of the features of this syndrome, indicating that it is the missing signal.[6] Leptin is produced exclusively in fat cells and the placenta, and signals the brain about the quantity of stored fat. The correlation between leptin and body fat is approximately 0.9. Leptin interacts with leptin receptors, which are widely distributed, including the brain. In most tissues, leptin receptors do not contain the complete intracellular signaling system, and may serve a binding or transport function. In tissues within the intracellular signaling domain, leptin binds to the extracellular receptor and activates intracellular signals that modulate a variety of bodily functions. Leptin modulates the expression of key hypothalamic peptides by reducing neuropeptide Y (NPY) and increasing α-MSH derived from pro-opiomelanocortin (POMC). The discovery of leptin generated a logarithmic increase in scientific work, as well as great intellectual excitement. This in turn stimulated a number of new approaches to developing better drugs for the treatment of obesity. It also served as a major piece of evidence that obesity is a serious disease that can be produced by genetic and molecular abnormalities.

The diabetes (db/db) mouse, fatty (Zucker) rat, and the Koletsky rat have defects in the leptin receptor. The db mouse is phenotypically identical to the ob mouse, indicating that obesity can be produced either by leptin deficiency or by genetic defects in the leptin receptor.[6] No human beings with obesity attributable to a leptin receptor defect have yet been described, but they probably exist.

The final two genes listed in Table 1 are for the Fat and Tubby mice. The Fat mouse lacks an effective carboxypeptidase E, which is involved in cleavage of many prohormones, including proinsulin. A family with a defect in a similar prohormone-converting enzyme and obesity was recently described.[7] The tub gene is associated with a number of neurologic defects. The tub gene may code for a phosphodiesterase and alter the function of hypothalamic neurons, thus producing a type of hypothalamic obesity.

A second approach to exploring the role of genetic factors in obesity is manipulation of the potential function of candidate genes for obesity, using transgenic animals.[1,2] Table 2 lists some of the transgenic models that have significant effects on food intake and body fat. The most striking result has been in the transgenic mouse in which the melanocortin-4 receptor is disabled.[8] This is the receptor where the agouti-signaling protein competes with α-MSH for receptor occupancy. Mice lacking the melanocortin-4 receptor become markedly obese, suggesting that a functional α-MSH receptor in the hypothalamus serves as an important inhibitory system on food intake and body fat level.

The second transgenic mouse of particular interest is one in which the serotonin-2C receptor is eliminated.[9] These animals show two defects. The first is an enhanced susceptibility to epilepsy and early death. The second is an increase in food intake and a variable degree of obe-

Table 2: Transgenic Models That Alter Body Fat

Models That Increase Body Fat

- Melanocortin-4 receptor knockout
- Glucocorticoid receptor antisense in brain
- CRH overexpression
- Uncoupling protein-1 knockout in brown adipose tissue
- Agouti-protein overexpression
- β_3-receptor knockout
- Glut-4 overexpression in fat
- Intracellular adhesion molecule-1 knockout
- Bombesin knockout

Models That Decrease Body Fat

- Lipoprotein lipase overexpression in muscle and cardiac tissue
- Uncoupling protein-1 overexpression in WAT and BAT
- Glycerol-3-phosphate dehydrogenase overexpression
- Protein kinase A knockout (RIIβ)
- Serotonin-2C knockout
- Glucokinase overexpression
- Agouti-related transcript overexpression

Models Without Effect

- Neuropeptide Y
- Y-5 receptor knockout
- Fatty acid binding protein knockout
- Glucagon-like peptide-1 knockout

Table 3: Heritability of Obesity

Types of Study	Heritability
Family studies	30%-50%
Adoption studies	10%-30%
Twins	50%-90%
Combined strategy	25%-40%

sity. Researchers believe the serotonin-2C receptor is the receptor through which serotonergic drugs reduce food intake.

A third transgenic model is one in which the hypothalamic glucocorticoid receptor is eliminated, thus preventing a feedback signal from serum glucocorticoids to suppress the adrenal gland. A slow and progressive obesity develops in these animals, suggesting the importance of glucocorticoids in the onset of obesity. One transgenic mouse has been surprising since it did not experience changes in food intake. This is the animal with NPY deficiency. NPY is one of the most potent stimulators of food intake, and we would expect that its removal would decrease feeding; however, this did not occur. Neither food intake nor body fat were affected by loss of NPY.[10]

Genetic Factors in Human Obesity

Three groups of studies were influential in pointing toward important genetic components of human obesity.[2] These were studies of twins, studies of adoptees, and studies of families. The estimates of heritability from these various approaches is summarized in Table 3. The heritability of obesity estimated from twin studies appeared to be high, from 0.6 to 0.9. From studies of adopted subjects and of twins reared apart, and from family studies, heritability levels appear to be between 0.2 and 0.4.[11]

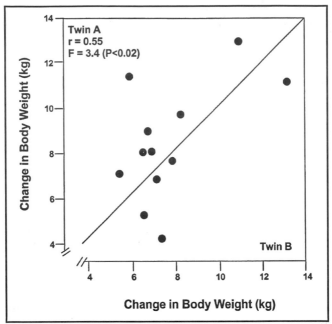

Figure 1: Effect on body fat of overfeeding identical twins.[12]
Copyright 1990, Massachusetts Medical Society. All rights reserved.

In addition to the overall heritability for weight, genetic epidemiologic studies have also established that metabolic rate, thermic response to food, and spontaneous physical activity show genetic components in their inheritance. The response to overfeeding of identical twins is one of the most persuasive studies (Figure 1). In this study, 12 pairs of identical twins were overfed for 100 days. Differences among twin pairs in average weight gain and fat storage were significant, but the differences between twins were considerably greater than the differences within pairs of twins. Thus, not only does current weight status have a strong inherited component, but also the metabolic processes underlying weight gain show strong genetic influences.[12]

Human obesity is associated with a number of defined genetic traits. At least 24 Mendelian disorders include obesity as a significant clinical feature.[2] Nine of these disorders are transmitted as autosomal dominant traits, 10 as autosomal recessive traits, and the remaining five are X-linked. Bardet-Biedl syndrome and Prader-Willi syndrome are probably the best-known examples of these traits (Chapter 5).[2]

Genome-wide searches using mapping techniques have been used to look for genes associated with obesity. The availability of numerous markers along the chromosomal map of the mouse and human being has made it possible to explore the obesity phenotype in animals that have different susceptibilities to becoming obese, and in human populations as well. More than a dozen different chromosome locations in animals have a high probability of showing a gene involved in the development of obesity. A similar strategy for examining the human genome is also underway. Linkage results in human studies demonstrate that more than six different linkage positions exist on different chromosomes. A number of genes involved in the development of human obesity clearly will be identified.[2] However, this search for genetic factors involved in obesity should not obscure the truth that environmental factors probably are more important. Human beings adapted in an environment of periodic food deficiency. The abundance that now confronts us, coupled with the associated sedentary lifestyle, are the main contributors to the worldwide epidemic of obesity outlined in Chapter 1. One of the clearest examples is the study of Pima Indians living their traditional agricultural lifestyle in Mexico, compared with Pima Indians living in Arizona. The mean BMI of Pima Indian women living in Arizona was 36 kg/m^2, compared with 25 kg/m^2 for matched women living in Mexico. The difference was less in men, although the Pima men living in Mexico had a body mass index (BMI) of 25 kg/m^2 compared with 31 kg/m^2 for those living in Arizona.[13] The

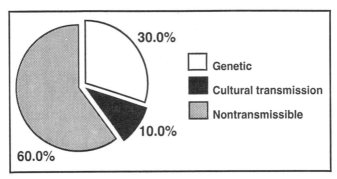

Figure 2: Genetic factors in obesity, using the subjects in the Quebec Family Study. Variance in body fat can be partitioned into genetic (30%), cultural (10%), and nontransmissible (60%) components.

relative role of various genetic, cultural, and environmental factors is presented in a pie chart (Figure 2). One of the leading scholars of the genetics of obesity put it this way: "It would not be surprising if behavioral differences would turn out to be more important than genetic differences in the etiology of overweight and obesity in technologically advanced societies."[11]

A Nutrient and Energy Model of Obesity

Obesity results from increased intake of energy or decreased expenditure of energy, as required by the first law of thermodynamics: *Change in body fat = Difference between intake and expenditure ($\Delta E = q\text{-}w$).* However, this simple relationship hides the important considerations involved in relating energy intake and energy expenditure. Figure 3 shows the first law of thermodynamics. Increasing energy intake (or, alternatively, decreasing energy expenditure) increases total body fat (top), but this alone does not explain the effect on fat distribution in the lower right, which is influenced by a variety of other variables, such as intrauterine growth,

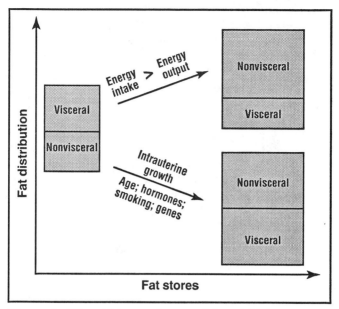

Figure 3: Effect of increasing total fat with the same or different fat distribution. Factors are shown above and below the arrows.

growth hormone, and reproductive hormones, among others.[14]

Overfeeding undoubtedly can increase body fat (Figure 1).[12] The remainder of this chapter examines the components of a feedback system shown in Figure 4. The controlled system consists of the cellular processes for energy expenditure and for the digestion, absorption, transport, and storage of nutrient fuels and their subsequent mobilization and use. The processes involved in this controlled system send afferent signals from the periphery to the central nervous system about deficits or surpluses of foods, or alterations in the rate of fuel use, as in exercise. The central nervous system, in turn, processes this afferent information and initiates metabolic and cognitive decisions

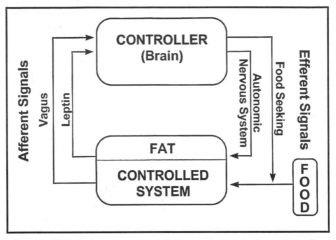

Figure 4: Feedback model for regulation of energy, fat, and nutrient balance.

about whether food is needed and, if so, when and where to get it. The controller also initiates processes through efferent controls of metabolism.[1]

The Controlled System
Energy Expenditure

Energy expenditure has several components (Figure 5).[15] Approximately two thirds of energy expenditure is used for 'basal' or 'resting' metabolism. This includes the energy involved in maintaining body temperature, in maintaining ionic gradients across cell membranes, in contracting smooth muscles for cardiac and gastrointestinal function, and for other metabolic storage and mobilization processes.

Figure 6 shows the relationship between energy expenditure and fat-free mass of subjects studied in a metabolic respiratory chamber.[16] Total daily energy expenditure or resting energy expenditure and fat-free mass are strongly related, implying that the fat-free mass contributes the

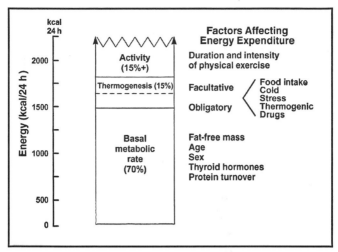

Figure 5: Components of energy expenditure.

chief component to this metabolic process. The energy expenditure expressed in this fashion in studies of the Pima Indians also has a strong familial relationship (Figure 7). These are consistent with the earlier observations on the familial components of resting metabolic rate obtained from studies of identical twins.[17] A low metabolic rate predicts the future development of obesity in this population, and this is supported in other studies.

Approximately 10% of energy expenditure is dissipated through the thermic responses to food (TEF). The TEF has two components: obligatory and facultative (Figure 5). The latter can be blocked by β-adrenergic blockade, suggesting that the sympathetic nervous system is important. A frequent question is whether a low thermic effect of food is related to the development of obesity. In a recent review, studies that were appropriately conducted clearly showed that obesity reduces the thermic effect of food.[18] Insulin resistance was a major component in this reduction in thermic response to food.

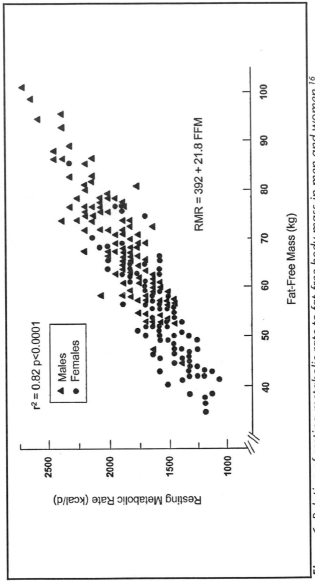

Figure 6: *Relation of resting metabolic rate to fat-free body mass in men and women.*[16]

48

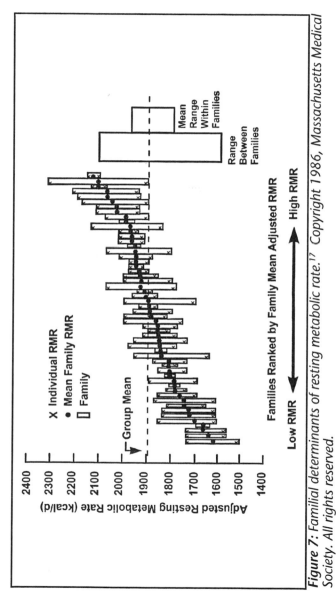

Figure 7: Familial determinants of resting metabolic rate.[17] Copyright 1986, Massachusetts Medical Society. All rights reserved.

49

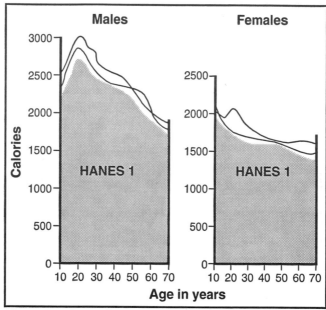

Figure 8: *Relationship of energy intake to age in both males and females. Data from three national surveys.*

If insulin resistance was present, the thermic effect was reduced. In small animals, brown adipose tissue, which is controlled by the sympathetic nervous system, is important in thermogenesis (heat production) in cold environments. This system is also important in maintaining body temperature in newborn mammals, including humans. The third component of energy expenditure is activity and exercise. The energy used for activity is related to body weight and the frequency, intensity, and duration of activity (Chapter 8). A number of studies suggest that overweight individuals spend less time in spontaneous physical activity. However, because they carry extra weight, the total amount of energy expended in physical activity may not be reduced.

Table 4: Caloric Value and Storage Capacity for the Four Major Macronutrients

Nutrient	Caloric Value (kcal/g)	Storage Capacity (kg)
Alcohol	7.1	0
Glucose	4.0	0.150
Protein	4.0	>10
Fat	9.2	>100

Energy Intake

Energy needed comes from food, and constitutes the other side of the energy equation.[19] Genetic influences may be less prominent here. Identical and nonidentical twins in a laboratory setting showed little ability to compensate for the energy differences in a milkshake consumed before lunch, and showed little genetic influence on this process.

Food intake has been measured in a number of cross-sectional surveys and in laboratory settings, which provide a snapshot of gender and age effects.[20] Figure 8 shows data from three surveys that yielded similar results. Total intake peaks in late adolescence and early adulthood, and then declines. At any age, men consume more calories than do women. The decrease in intake with age has been documented in longitudinal studies. Middle-aged men had a decline of 450 kcal/d over 10 years.[21] The rise in body weight over these 10 years indicates that energy expenditure must have fallen even more. The intake of energy reported from dietary surveys probably underestimates actual energy expenditure. The use of doubly labeled water to measure total energy expenditure has allowed for comparison of energy from food intake records with total energy expenditure. Normal-weight individuals underreport

Table 5: Randomized Dietary Fat Intervention Studies Without Energy Restriction[23]

Investigators	Intervention group (n)	Change in % dietary fat
Puska et al (1983)[24]	35	39 → 23
Sheppard et al (1991)[25]	184	39.2 → 20.9
Hunninghake et al (1993)[26]	97	41 → 26
Kazim et al (1993)[27]	34	36 → 18
Levitsky & Strupp (1994)[28]	28	37 → 27
Shah et al (1994)[29]	47	33.8 → 21.0

by an average of 20%, and overweight individuals under-report by 30% or more.[15,22] The underreporting of energy intake yielded the erroneous concept that obese individuals often did not eat more than lean ones. The rise in total energy expenditure with body weight as measured by a variety of methods (Figure 6) means that overweight individuals, on average, eat more. If they continue to gain weight, they continue to eat more than their body needs for fuel.

The four nutrients that provide the sources of energy have very different energy values and storage capacity in the body (Table 4). Alcohol has little or no storage capacity. The storage capacity for carbohydrate is small, and these nutrients must be completely or largely metabolized quickly after ingestion.[30] The large storage capacity for fat, and the relationship of fat intake to overall changes in body weight in the obesity epidemic, have targeted dietary fat as a component that might be reduced.

The nature of the diet is involved in the development of obesity. The association of a 'Western' diet with more than 30% of calories from fat is associated with increasing weight in Japanese who migrated from Japan to Ha-

Intervention period	Mean weight loss (kg)	Rate (g/d)
6 weeks	0.7	17
9 months	3.2	18
9 weeks	1.4	22
3 months	3.4	38
6 weeks	0.9	22
6 months	4.4	24

waii and California.[23] The percentage of Japanese children in Japan who are obese has also risen as the percentage of fat in the Japanese diet has risen.

Conversely, dietary intervention studies using low-fat diets have shown small but modest decreases in body weight, averaging 0.7 to 4.4 kg. Several of these are summarized in Table 5, adapted from a review by Lissner et al.[23] These effects suggest that modestly lowering dietary fat may not much affect obesity once it has developed, but this is true of other treatments as well, indicating that it is better to prevent than to treat obesity. Preventing the rise in dietary fat in the diet of developing countries, on the other hand, may prevent or slow the epidemic of obesity.

The food supply in the United States has changed steadily. Through the mid 20th century, consumption of dietary fat continued to rise, replacing starches in the diet. Consumption of refined sugar also rose, and consumption of fruits and vegetables declined. Over the past 25 years, fat intake stabilized and then began to decline. This decline occurred as the prevalence of overweight rose slowly, and then exploded. If the fat intake had not declined, the epidemic of obesity might be worse.

Two other features of the food supply also may be important in the epidemic of obesity. Between the 1930s and 1990s, the energy per person available from the food supply increased by about 500 kcal/d. Net storage of 20 kcal/d, requiring an additional 30 kcal/d of total energy to allow for metabolic costs of storage, would be required to account for an increase in body weight of 10 kg in 10 years, assuming that this increase in weight is 70% fat.

The energy density of the diet is the other factor. When energy density of the food supply is reduced, ie, fewer kcal/g of food, a larger mass (weight) of food must be eaten to provide the same amount of energy. Several studies suggest that consumption of food may be partly regulated by the mass or weight consumed. A more energy-dense diet would thus tend to be 'overconsumed.'[19] Reduction of energy density in the processed food supply may thus provide a strategy to reduce energy intake as an approach to obesity.

Metabolized fuels are involved in the development of obesity. The mixture of fuels used by the body can be measured from the ratio of carbon dioxide production to oxygen use (respiratory quotient [RQ] or respiratory exchange ratio). The amount of oxygen needed to metabolize daily food, and the carbon dioxide produced during this oxidation, are related to the amount of fat and carbohydrate in the diet. The ratio of CO_2 formed to O_2 needed to metabolize fat and carbohydrate in the diet is the food quotient (FQ). If the RQ is higher than the FQ, carbohydrate is being oxidized and body stores of glycogen are being depleted. Because carbohydrate reserves are limited, one of two metabolic strategies are available. First, the body can reduce the use of carbohydrate, which equally increases the oxidation of fat to redress the balance. Alternatively, the individual can eat more food to provide carbohydrate for daily needs, and store the excess fat energy in fat cells. The first strategy is preferred because it prevents depletion of carbohydrate

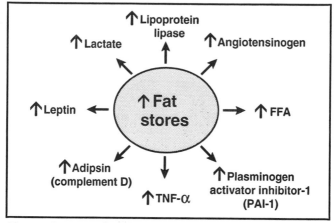

Figure 9: Fat cell as an endocrine cell. TNF-α = tumor necrosis factor-alpha.

stores and the development of obesity. If it fails, the ingestion of extra carbohydrate results in obesity. One prediction from this reasoning is that a high RQ precedes or predicts obesity, and this has been found in studies of the Pima Indians.

Metabolic Features of the Controlled System

Insulin and the pancreas. One characteristic of the controlled system in the obese body is hyperinsulinemia, which results from increased insulin secretion by the pancreas. Insulin secretion is increased in direct relationship to the degree of excess fat, and may be a signal for leptin production by fat cells. The portal vein delivers secreted insulin to the liver. The increased insulin in the liver is partially degraded, and the remainder enters the peripheral circulation. In the liver, insulin signals for increased triglyceride secretion packaged in very-low-density lipoprotein particles, and for decreased HDL cholesterol production. In the peripheral circulation, the increased insulin and possibly tumor necrosis factor-α (TNF-α), a

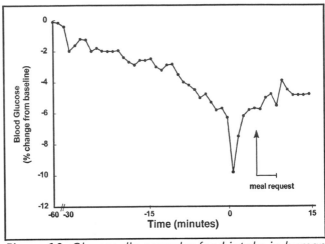

Figure 10: Glucose dip precedes food intake in human volunteers.[32]

cytokine from fat cells, induce insulin resistance. This insulin resistance is shown by the decreased response to insulin in muscle and adipose tissue.

Skeletal muscle. Uptake of fatty acids by muscle is higher in muscles from obese subjects than from lean ones in the basal state, but insulin does not stimulate fatty acid uptake in muscles of obese subjects as it does in lean individuals exposed to insulin. In addition to insulin resistance, obese individuals show a decrease in type I insulin-responsive oxidative fibers and an increase in type II fibers.

Fat cells. Adipocytes are enlarged in obese individuals, and the total number of fat cells may be increased in the massively obese.[1,6] Fat cells store triglyceride, but also are endocrine cells (Figure 9). Enlarged fat cells have a higher turnover of triglyceride and secrete more leptin.[4,6] They also secrete a variety of peptides, including lipoprotein lipase, TNF-α, angiotensinogen, and complement D (adipsin).

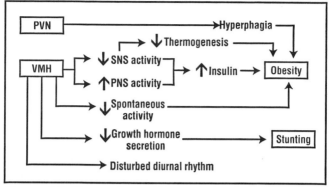

Figure 11: Comparison of hypothalamic lesions in the paraventricular nucleus (PVN) and ventromedial hypothalamus (VMH). PNS = parasympathetic nervous system; SNS = sympathetic nervous system.

Liver. The liver enlarges in relationship to the degree of obesity. In very large individuals, a fatty liver may develop because of the high flux of fatty acids.

Afferent Signals

Fat cells. The controlled system generates a number of messages that tell the brain about the state of the body[1] (Figures 4 and 9). The first of these is leptin, which is produced exclusively in fat cells.[4,6] It strongly correlates with body fat ($r=0.9$). Leptin can reduce food intake and enhance the activity of the sympathetic nervous system in rodents and nonhuman primates. Leptin deficiency has recently been reported in two children who were cousins.[5] Circulating leptin levels are higher in women than men, and have a pulsatile secretion and diurnal rhythm. The nocturnal rise in leptin is lower in overweight individuals than in controls.

Gastrointestinal tract. The concept that the gastrointestinal (GI) tract is involved in signaling hunger and satiety was formulated more than 100 years ago. This concept is

Table 6: Monoamines and Peptides That Affect Feeding

Effect on Food Intake

Decrease	Increase
• Norepinephrine (α_2)	• Norepinephrine (α_1; β_2)
• Neuropeptide Y	• Serotonin (5-HT$_{1B}$;5-HT$_{2C}$)
• Opioids (dynorphin)	• Cholecystokinin
• Melanin-concentrating hormone	• Melanocyte-stimulating hormone (α-MSH)
• Growth hormone releasing hormone	• Corticotropin-releasing hormone/urocortin
• Galanin	• Glucagon (GLP-1)
• β-Casomorphin	• Enterostatin
	• Leptin

borne out in many people's daily experience. Gastric distention can signal satiety, and gastric contractions can signal hunger. As the stomach expands during eating, the distention may activate vagal fibers to produce satiety. Conversely, the well-known queasiness or crampy stomach that occurs when the stomach is 'empty' is associated with hunger for many people.

Vagus nerve. The vagal afferent system from the gastrointestinal tract to the brain is a major pathway for the afferent signals generated in the GI tract. The reduction in food intake produced by cholecystokinin (CCK), a gastrointestinal peptide, and enterostatin, which is derived from pancreatic procolipase, both depend on an intact vagus nerve to relay their information to the brain.[31]

Nutrient signals. Nutrients absorbed from the gastrointestinal tract may also serve as signals to the brain about hunger and satiety. A small dip in plasma glucose, approximately 10%, precedes more than half the meals in experiments in animals,[27] and appears to be important in humans as well. This glucose dip reflects the stimulation of insulin release that precedes the drop in glucose. The release of insulin probably is related to a vagal-afferent stimulation of insulin output. The studies of Campfield et al suggest that the pattern of change in glucose is being detected, because preventing the drop in glucose delays the onset of the next meal (Figure 10).[32]

Sensory signals. Messages from the periphery reach the brain through blood or nerves. Information from visual and auditory stimuli, as well as from the taste and smell of food or other environmental elements, are relayed to the hindbrain and processed in the nucleus of the tractus solitarius. Humoral messages from leptin and possibly glucose and amino acids may be evaluated after transport across the blood-brain barrier, or in those restricted regions of the brain where the blood barrier is absent.

Controller

Anatomy. Within the brain, a variety of messages are involved in the control of food intake.[33] At least four anatomic regions seem important in processing information about food and relating it to body weight. The first of these is the nucleus of the tractus solitarius in the hindbrain, where vagal information and information about taste and smell may be integrated. The second area is the VMH, where much information is processed. When this region is destroyed, profound obesity develops in all species studied. In animals with VMH lesions, food intake increases, the parasympathetic nervous system becomes more active, and the sympathetic nervous system becomes less active. The effects of lesions in the paraventricular nucleus (PVN) and ventromedial nucleus (VMN) are shown in Figure 11.

The PVN modulates feeding. Prevention of hyperphagia in animals with PVN lesions prevents the obesity. Hyperphagia, however, is not required for obesity in animals with a VMN lesion, because damage to this region alters the activity of the autonomic nervous system and leads to obesity. Selected regions of the amygdala (central nucleus) may also be important in modulating feeding, through connections to either the PVN, the VMH, or elsewhere. Finally, damage to the lateral hypothalamus may decrease feeding and lower body weight.

Monoamine neurotransmitters. A variety of monoamines are involved as neurotransmitters or neuromodulators of feeding and energy expenditure (Table 6). Norepinephrine (NE) acts on α_1-adrenoceptors in the PVN to decrease food intake. An α_2-adrenoceptor in the PVN is involved in the stimulation of food intake by NE. Finally, stimulation of β_2-adrenoceptors reduces food intake.

Serotonin acts on seven families of receptors to modulate a variety of functions, including food intake. Stimulation of the 5-HT_{1A} receptor acutely stimulates food intake, but this response rapidly attenuates. Reduction in food intake by serotonin probably occurs by action on the 5-HT_{2C} receptor. This conclusion is supported by the finding that mice whose 5-HT_{2C} receptors have been eliminated show weight gain.[9] Serotonergic drugs probably act through this 5-HT_{2C} receptor. In animals, stimulation of serotonin receptors in the hypothalamus primarily reduces fat intake. Reduction in fat intake also appears to be predominant with serotonergic drugs used clinically.

Peptide neuromodulators. The list of peptides that stimulate or suppress food intake continues to grow.[1,33] NPY is one of the most potent stimulators of food intake. Chronic injection or infusion of NPY increases food intake and body weight. Thus, the transgenic mouse that did not make NPY and had perfectly normal control of food intake and body weight was surprising.[10] Nonetheless, NPY remains one of the potent stimulators of feeding in NPY-deficient and intact animals. In addition to stimulating food intake, NPY primarily stimulates carbohydrate intake. Antagonists to one of the NPY receptors (NPY Y-5) are being evaluated as a site for new drugs. Dynorphin, melanin-concentrating hormone (MCH), and growth hormone releasing hormone (GHRH) also stimulate food intake.

The list of inhibitory peptides is much longer,[1,33] but separating effects on food intake from other effects, such as aversion to food or stimulation of alternate behaviors (eg, sleeping, exploring, drinking), often is difficult. However, some of these peptides appear to be biologically important in modulating feeding. The first of these is CCK, which decreases food intake centrally as well as peripherally. Drugs modulating CCK receptors also affect food intake, reinforcing its importance. Enterostatin is a particularly interesting peptide because it is derived from a proenzyme in the gastrointestinal tract, procolipase, which is conserved across many species.[31] Enterostatin is a pentapeptide that reduces food intake whether given peripherally or into the brain. It specifically reduces fat intake and affects neither carbohydrate nor protein intake. Thus, along with serotonin, enterostatin is a potent nutrient-specific inhibitor of fat intake.

Corticotropin-releasing hormone (CRH) or a similar peptide, urocortin, may act through CRH-2 receptors to reduce food intake, and to stimulate the sympathetic nervous system and inhibit the parasympathetic nervous system. Melanocyte-stimulating hormone (α-MSH) may be another important modulator of feeding, because damage to the melanocortin-4 receptor in the hypothalamus leads to massive obesity.[8] Glucagon-like peptide-1, the 6-29 amino acid segment of glucagon, depresses food intake when injected centrally, but because mice that make no glucagon-like peptide-1 have normal body weight and normal food intake, its physiologic role is unclear.

Table 7: Reciprocal Relationship of Food Intake and Sympathetic Activity

Experimental Maneuver	Changes in Food Intake	Changes in Sympathetic Activity
Lesion in the hypothalamus		
VMN/PVN	↑	↓
LH	↓	↑
Peptides - group 1	↑	↓
(NPY; GAL; opioids)		
Peptides - group 2	↓	↑
(CRH; BBS; CCK)		
Chemicals - group 1	↑	↓
(2-DG; NE)		
Chemicals - group 2	↓	↑
(Fenfluramine; 5HT)		

VMN = ventromedial nucleus; PVN = paraventricular nucleus;
LH = lateral hypothalamus; NPY = neuropeptide Y;
GAL = galanin; CRH = corticotropin-releasing hormone;
BBS = bombesin; CCK = cholecystokinin;
2DG = 2-deoxy-D-glucose; NE = norepinephrine;
5HT = serotonin

Ion channels. At least two ion channels in the medial hypothalamus modulate feeding. Activation of the chloride channel by γ-aminobutyric acid (GABA) increases food intake, but similar treatment in the lateral hypothalamic area reduces food intake. Potassium-channel antagonists reduce food intake, whereas potassium-channel openers increase feeding.

Efferent Controls

The transducers of afferent information modulate several efferents that attenuate food intake and internal metabolic processes. The first process is the search for and ingestion of food. Food seeking and ingestion are complex, involving both internal signals and external information. Time of day, social context, and options or requirements for alternate activities all influence food intake. In addition, motor systems identify the source and acceptability of food. Once ingested, food enters the controlled system for digestion, absorption, distribution to various tissues, storage, and metabolism.

The second efferent control is over the autonomic nervous system. Vagal efferent fibers 'alert' the GI tract and pancreas that food is about to be eaten. This 'cephalic'-phase release of insulin slightly increases insulin secretion and provides information to the stomach, intestine, and other tissues about the imminent arrival of food.

Food ingestion also activates the efferent sympathetic nervous system, which is involved in the thermic response to food. Experimental studies show that the activity of the peripheral sympathetic nerves supplying thermogenic tissues and food intake are reciprocally related. There is a strong, robust relationship between activity of the sympathetic nervous system and food intake. This relationship applies to lesions, peptides, and drugs (Table 7). The data from the Pima Indians show that a low sympathetic activity predicts obesity in humans.[34] One implication of this is that β_3-adrenergic receptors may mediate satiety signals. Stimulation of β_3-receptors with β_3-agonists indeed acutely reduces food intake.[35] Animals that lack β_3-receptors in white adipose tissue do not reduce food intake in response to β_3-agonists.[35]

The third efferent system is adrenal glucocorticoids. Cushing's disease with increased glucocorticoid production is associated with central obesity (Chapter 4), and Addison's disease, or adrenal insufficiency, is associated with weight loss and loss of body fat. In the absence of adrenal glucocorticoids, none of the experimental animal models became obese.[1] Animals with leptin deficiency or VMH lesions depend on glucocorticoids for the expression of obesity. This may be attributable to the inhibition of sympathetic nervous system activity.

Body Fat Distribution

The second component of the model in Figure 3 is the distribution of body fat between visceral and subcutaneous compartments and within different subcutaneous areas.[36] Gonadal steroids obviously are very important in this process. At the onset of puberty, males become more muscular and less fat, whereas females increase their body fat relative to muscle mass. These differences persist throughout life and are reflected in the typical male and female fat distribution and differences in body composition. With aging, body composition changes with increasing visceral and total fat. Hormonal factors may be important in this shift. With age, both testosterone and growth hormone decline, and this may be important in the rise in visceral fat with age, particularly in men. In women, higher testosterone levels usually are associated with increased visceral fat. The decline in growth hormone and the loss of estrogen during menopause thus may be involved in the relatively rapid increase in visceral fat in the postmenopausal years.

Activity of the hypothalamic-pituitary-adrenal (HPA) axis has been proposed as one mechanism for the development of visceral fat.[37] A recent study suggested that central obesity may be a form of Cushing's disease of the omentum, resulting from failure to inactivate cortisol to cortisone. The enzyme (11-β-hydroxysteroid dehydrogenase) involved in this transformation was higher in omental fat than in subcutaneous stromal fat, and converted inactive cortisone into cortisol.[38] Such a mechanism could expose omental fat cells to higher levels of cortisol and enhance the function of these visceral fat cells.[32]

References

1.   Bray GA, York DA: Obesity. In: Jefferson WS, Cherrington A, eds. *Handbook of Physiology*. Washington, DC, American Physiology Society, 1998, in press.

2.   Chagnon YC, Perusse L, Bouchard C: The human obesity gene map: the 1997 update. *Obes Res* 1998;6:76-92.

3.   Bultman SJ, Michaud EJ, Woychik RP: Molecular characterization of the mouse agouti locus. *Cell* 1992;71:1195-1294.

4.   Zhang YY, Proenca R, Maffei M, et al: Positional cloning of the mouse obese gene and its human homologue. *Nature* 1994;372:425-432.

5.   Montague CT, Farooqi IS, Whitehead JP, et al: Congenital leptin deficiency is associated with severe early-onset obesity in humans. *Nature* 1997;387:903-908.

6.   Bray GA, York DA: Clinical review 90: Leptin and clinical medicine: a new piece in the puzzle of obesity. *J Clin Endocrinol Metab* 1997;82:2771-2776.

7.   Jackson RS, Creemers JW, Ohagi S, et al: Obesity and impaired prohormone processing associated with mutations in the human prohormone convertase 1 gene. *Nat Genet* 1997;16:303-306.

8.   Huszar D, Lynch CA, Fairchild-Huntress V, et al: Targeted disruption of the melanocortin-4 receptor results in obesity in mice. *Cell* 1997;88:131-141.

9.   Tecott LH, Sun LM, Akana SF, et al: Eating disorder and epilepsy in mice lacking the 5-HT$_2$ serotonin receptors. *Nature* 1995;374:542-546.

10.   Erickson JC, Clegg KE, Palmiter RD: Sensitivity to leptin and susceptibility to seizures of mice lacking neuropeptide Y. *Nature* 1996;381:415-421.

11.   Bouchard C: Genetics of obesity: overview and research direction. In: Bouchard CB, ed. *The Genetics of Obesity*. Boca Raton, CRC Press, 1994, pp 223-233.

12.   Bouchard C, Tremblay A, Despres JP, et al: The response to long-term overfeeding in identical twins. *N Engl J Med* 1990; 322:1477-1482.

13. Ravussin E, Valencia ME, Esparza J, et al: Effects of a traditional lifestyle on obesity in Pima Indians. Diabetes Care 1994;17:1067-1074.

14. Fried SK, Russell CD: Diverse roles of adipose tissue in the regulation of systemic metabolism and energy balance. In: Bray GA, Bouchard C, James WP, eds. *Handbook of Obesity*. New York, Marcel Dekker, 1997, pp 397-414.

15. Schutz Y, Jequier E: Resting energy expenditure, thermic effect of food, and total energy expenditure. In: Bray GA, Bouchard C, James WP, eds. *Handbook of Obesity*. New York, Marcel Dekker, 1997, pp 443-456.

16. Ravussin E, Lillioja S, Anderson TE, et al: Determinants of 24-hour energy expenditure in man. Methods and results using a respiratory chamber. *J Clin Invest* 1986;78:1568-1578.

17. Bogardus C, Lillioja S, Ravussin E, et al: Familial dependence of the resting metabolic rate. *N Engl J Med* 1986;315:96-100.

18. de Jonge L, Bray GA: The thermic effect of food and obesity: a critical review. *Obes Res* 1997;5:622-631.

19. Blundell JE, Stubbs RJ: Diet composition and the control of food intake in humans. In: Bray GA, Bouchard C, James WP, eds. *Handbook of Obesity*. New York, Marcel Dekker, 1997, pp 243-272.

20. Bray GA, Gray DS: Obesity. Part II—Treatment. *West J Med* 1988;149:555-571.

21. Kromhout D: Changes in energy and macronutrients in 871 middle-aged men during 10 years of follow-up (the Zutphen study). *Am J Clin Nutr* 1983;37:287-294.

22. Schoeller DA, Fjeld CR: Human energy metabolism: what have we learned from the doubly labeled water method? *Annu Rev Nutr* 1991;11:355-373.

23. Lissner L, Heitmann BL: Dietary fat and obesity: evidence from epidemiology. *Eur J Clin Nutr* 1995;49:79-90.

24. Puska P, Iacono JM, Nissinen A, et al: Controlled, randomised trial of the effect of dietary fat on blood pressure. *Lancet* 1983;1:1-5.

25. Sheppard L, Kristal AR, Kushi LH: Weight loss in women participating in a randomized trial of low-fat diets. *Am J Clin Nutr* 1991;54:821-828.

26. Hunninghake DB, Stein EA, Dujovne CA, et al: The efficacy of intensive dietary therapy alone or combined with lovastatin in

outpatients with hypercholesterolemia. *N Engl J Med* 1993; 328:1213-1219.

27. Kasim SE, Martino S, Kim PN, et al: Dietary and anthropometric determinants of plasma lipoproteins during a long-term low-fat diet in healthy women. *Am J Clin Nutr* 1993;57:146-153.

28. Levitsky DA, Strupp BJ: Imprecise control of food intake on low fat diets. In: Fernstrom JD, Miller GD, eds. *Appetite and Body Weight Regulation: Sugar, Fat and Macronutrients.* Boca Raton, CRC Press, 1994.

29. Shah M, McGovern P, French S, et al: Comparison of a low-fat, ad libitum complex-carbohydrate diet with a low-energy diet in moderately obese women. *Am J Clin Nutr* 1994;59:980-984.

30. Jebb SA, Prentice AM, Goldberg GR, et al: Changes in macronutrient balance during over- and underfeeding assessed by 12-d continuous whole-body calorimetry. *Am J Clin Nutr* 1996;64: 259-266.

31. Erlanson-Albertsson C, York D: Enterostatin—a peptide regulating fat intake. *Obes Res* 1997;5:360-372.

32. Campfield LA, Smith FJ: Blood glucose dynamics and the control of meal initiation: a pattern detection and recognition theory. *Physiol Rev* 1998, in press.

33. Leibowitz SF, Hoebel BG: Behavioral neuroscience of obesity. In: Bray GA, Bouchard C, James WP, eds. *Handbook of Obesity.* New York, Marcel Dekker, 1997, pp 313-358.

34. Tataranni PA, Young JB: A low sympathoadrenal activity is associated with body weight gain and development of central adiposity in Pima Indian men. *Obes Res* 1997;5:341-347.

35. Susulic VS, Frederich RC, Lawitts J, et al: Targeted disruption of the β_3-adrenergic receptor gene. *J Biol Chem* 1995; 270:29483-29492.

36. Arner P: Adipose tissue as a storage organ. In: Bray GA, Bouchard C, James WP, eds. *Handbook of Obesity.* New York, Marcel Dekker, 1997, pp 379-396.

37. Bjorntorp P: Visceral obesity: a "civilization syndrome". *Obes Res* 1993;1:206-222.

38. Bujalska IJ, Kumar S, Stewart PM: Does central obesity reflect "Cushing's disease of the omentum"? *Lancet* 1997;349:1210-1213.

Chapter 3

Health Hazards Associated With Overweight

......................Leave gourmandizing,
Know the grave doth gape for thee
Thrice wider than for other men.

— Shakespeare
Henry IV
Act V, Scene 5, 54-55

Overweight patients are at risk for developing a number of medical, social, and psychologic disabilities (Figure 1). The spectrum includes a range of medical and behavior problems.

The effects of excess weight on morbidity and mortality have been known for more than 2,000 years. Hippocrates recognized that "sudden death is more common in those who are naturally fat than in the lean." Much literature has addressed this subject over the past 50 years; additional reading provides more detail.[1-7] The diseases associated with overweight also are responsible for significant health-care costs. In this cost-conscious era, several analyses of health costs related to obesity have been done around the world. Between 3% and 7% of total health-care costs can be attributed to overweight. The direct cost by various disease categories for the United States is shown in Table 1.[8]

Overweight also increases use of the health-care system. In a study of health-care expenditures, individuals

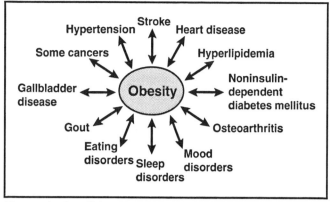

Figure 1: Conditions associated with obesity.

at the extremes of body mass index (BMI) had the highest expenditures, and individuals in the middle of the BMI range (26-27 kg/m^2) had the lowest probability of health-care expenditures. The probability of health-care expenditures increased significantly at both extremes of

Table 1: Cost of Obesity in the United States, 1995[8]

Disease	Direct Cost (in Billions)
Diabetes mellitus	$32.4
Coronary heart disease	$7.0
Osteoarthritis	$4.3
Hypertension	$3.2
Gallbladder disease	$2.6
Colon cancer	$1.0
Breast cancer	$0.84
Endometrial cancer	$0.29

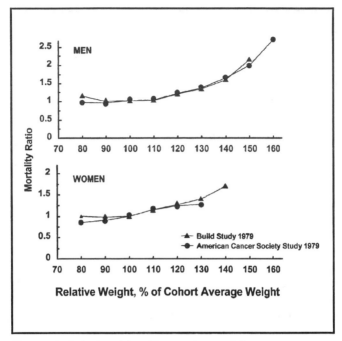

Figure 2: Relationship of increasing weight to excess mortality in three large studies.[15]

BMI for subjects with positive baseline expenditures, compared with subjects without baseline expenditures. BMI was associated with the annual number of inpatient days, number and costs of outpatient visits, costs of outpatient pharmacy, and laboratory and total costs in a large health-maintenance organization.[9] Mean annual costs were 25% higher in participants with a BMI between 30 and 35 kg/m^2, and were 44% higher in those with a BMI above 35 kg/m^2, compared with individuals with a BMI of 20 to 25 kg/m^2.[9] In the Swedish Obesity Study, obese subjects were 2.3 to 2.7 times more likely to draw a disability pension as were the normal population.[10] Prevention of conversion from preoverweight to clinically overweight status, or reversal of status if the patient gains weight, would have far-reaching economic implications.

Effects of Overweight, Body Fat Distribution, Weight Gain, and Sedentary Lifestyle on Mortality

Increased Body Weight

Increased overweight is associated with increased risk of death. The life insurance industry has been key in making the public aware of the relationship between increased weight and higher death rates. Four large studies, the Life Insurance Build Study of 1979,[11] the American Cancer Society study,[12] the Norwegian population study,[13] and the Nurses' Health Study,[14] as well as many smaller epidemiologic studies,[7] support these findings. The similarity of the two sets of life insurance data and the American Cancer Society study is shown in Figure 2.[15] As noted in a critical review of the studies, the effects of smoking or early deaths were not controlled. When smokers were eliminated in a 12-year follow-up of nurses, increasing BMI only resulted in a graded increase in mortality, which became significant at a BMI between 27 and 29.9 kg/m^2 (Figure 3).[14]

A very graphic demonstration of the continuing impact of excess weight is a 35-year follow-up of inductees into the Danish army. Overweight men with a BMI >31 kg/m^2 had a shorter life span than did men in the normal range of BMI (Figure 4).[16] The two lines continued to separate over time. The obvious impact of excess weight on increased mortality has not always been found in epidemiologic studies. In an analysis of the studies, which either did or did not show an effect of overweight on mortality, Sjostrom found that large studies with more than 10,000 participants, and smaller studies with a long-term follow-up of more than 15 years, almost unanimously found a relationship between BMI and mortality.[7]

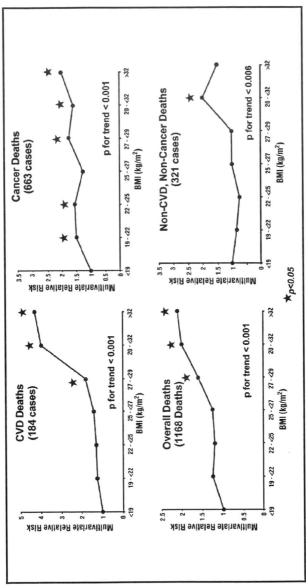

Figure 3: *Relationship of BMI to risk of death and several causes of death in the Nurses' Health Study.*[14]

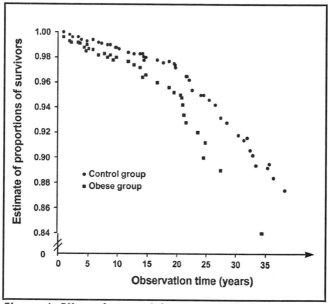

Figure 4: *Effect of overweight on survival after examination for induction in the Danish Army.*[16]

Figure 5 shows the relationship between BMI and the increasing relative risk to mortality, along with risk associated with two other risk factors: hypertension and hypercholesterolemia.[17] Areas of low risk, moderate risk, and high risk are demarcated by vertical dotted lines. Blood pressure, cholesterol, and overweight are risk factors that produce diseases through long-term exposure to elevated risk factors. Renal failure, heart failure, and stroke result from prolonged elevations in blood pressure. Atherosclerosis, with coronary and cerebrovascular occlusion, results from elevated cholesterol. Diabetes, gallbladder disease, heart failure, and some kinds of cancer are most strongly associated with overweight. Chronic exposure to elevated risk factors produces the disease states.

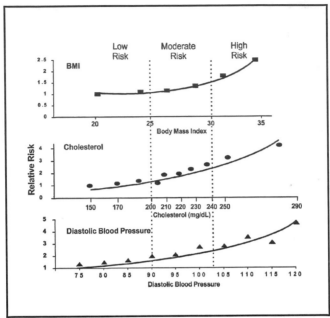

Figure 5: Relative risk associated with body weight, cholesterol, and blood pressure. All three risk factors show a curvilinear increase as the value rises. The areas of low, moderate, and high risk are identified by vertical dotted lines.

Several other studies also are instructive. In the Nurses' Health Study, deaths from cardiovascular disease and cancer deaths were the chief sources of increased mortality among 114,868 nurses observed over 13 years of follow-up.[15] Among 8,800 7th-Day Adventist men followed for 26 years, those with a BMI greater than 27.5 kg/m² had a 2-fold risk of death from all causes, and a 3.3-fold risk of dying from coronary heart disease, compared with 7th-Day Adventist men with a BMI <22.3 kg/m². Interestingly, the mean age at death of men with a BMI below 22.3 kg/m² was 80.5 years, compared with 75.8 years in the 7th-Day Adventist men whose BMI was greater than 27.5 kg/m².

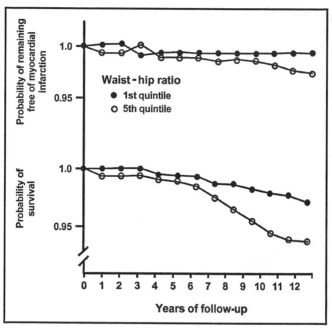

Figure 6: *Relationship of waist circumference divided by hip circumference to overall mortality and risk of myocardial infarction in the Gothenburg study.[19]*

The Harvard Alumni Study also showed important effects of overweight on mortality. Among 19,292 male Harvard alumni, average age 46.6 years, those who had a BMI above 26 kg/m² showed a 1.67-fold increase in mortality, compared with those who were followed for the same 27 years but whose BMI was less than 22.5 kg/m². The lowest mortality in the Harvard Alumni study was among men weighing an average of 20% below the mean for U.S. men of comparable age.

In 1993, 1.25 million deaths from natural causes occurred in American men and women aged 35 to 74, whose BMI was greater than 21 kg/m². Of this 1.25 million,

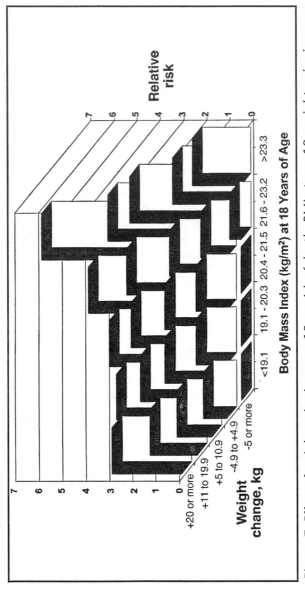

Figure 7: *Effect of weight gain since age 18 on risk of death. BMI at age 18, weight gain since age 18, and relative risk of mortality in subjects from the Nurses' Health Study are plotted.*[20]

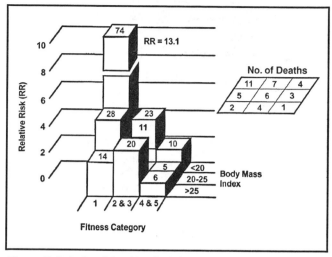

Figure 8: *Relationship of level of physical activity to mortality.*[21]

325,000 deaths could be attributed to overweight.[18] Some 77,315 deaths out of 406,923 deaths from coronary heart disease, and 34,413 deaths out of 55,110 deaths from diabetes, could be attributed to obesity. More than 50% of all-cause mortality among the 18 million women and 16.7 million men in the United States aged 20 to 74 with a BMI of greater than 30 kg/m^2 can be attributed to overweight.

Regional Fat Distribution

Regional fat distribution also is important in the risk of death.[2,3] The life insurance industry first noted this at the beginning of the 20th century. This theme was picked up again after World War II, when researchers noted that obese individuals with an android or male distribution of body fat were at higher risk for diabetes and heart disease than were those with a gynoid or female type of obesity. However, clinical and epidemiologic work in the 1980s

Table 2: Relative Risk of Health Problems Associated With Obesity in Developed Countries[22]

Greatly increased (relative risk >3)	Moderately increased (relative risk 2-3)	Slightly increased (relative risk 1-2)
Diabetes	Coronary heart disease	Cancer (breast cancer in post-menopausal women, endo-metrial cancer, colon cancer)
Gallbladder disease	Osteoarthritis (knees)	Reproductive hormone abnormalities
Hypertension	Hyperuricemia and gout	Polycystic ovary syndrome
Dyslipidemia		Impaired fertility
Insulin resistance		Low back pain from obesity
Breathlessness		Increased anesthetic risk
Sleep apnea		Fetal defects from maternal obesity

convinced the world of the relationship between body fat distribution and risk of excess mortality. The data in Figure 6 are from the Gothenburg longitudinal study.[19] In this study, central obesity was evaluated using the ratio of the waist circumference divided by the hip circumference (WHR). Women and men with the highest degree of central obesity had higher death rates than did those with the least central fat. Women in the highest quintile of central obesity had mortality rates similar to those of men in the lowest quintile of central obesity, suggesting that the higher mortality rates in men may be related to the effects of differences in fat distribution. Differences in central fatness will be used, like BMI, in evaluating the risk of overweight (Chapter 5). In addition to excess mortality, the risk of heart attacks, diabetes, and some forms of cancer was increased by central fatness.

Weight Gain

In addition to overweight and central fatness, the amount of weight gain after age 18 to 20 also predicts mortality. This is clearly illustrated in the Nurses' Health Study and the Health Professionals Study, in which a graded increase in mortality from heart disease is associated with increasing degrees of weight gain (Figure 7).[20] A gain of more than 10 kg indicates a higher level of increased risk. Weight gain in men after age 20 in the Health Professionals Study showed a similar relationship.

Sedentary Lifestyle

A sedentary lifestyle is a final important component in the relationship of excess mortality to overweight. A sedentary lifestyle by itself increases the mortality rates from all causes, as shown in Figure 8,[21] and part of this may relate to increased fatness and its comorbid correlates.

Intentional Weight Loss

If overweight increases risk of mortality, then we would anticipate that intentional weight loss would reduce it. A definitive demonstration of this prediction is not available, but several studies suggest that intentional weight loss does reduce risk. Weight loss reduces blood pressure, improves abnormal lipid levels, and reduces risk of diabetes.[23] Patients treated for obesity with gastric operations have been reported to have lower rates of death. A

Table 3:	Effect by Gender and Ethnic Group of Health Risks[26]		
	Age-Adjusted Odds Ratio for BMI >40 kg/m²		
	Men		
Disease	White	African American	Mexican American
Diabetes (NIDDM)	24.3	5.1	12.2
Hypertension	6.8	14.4	22.5
Gallbladder disease	12.5	—	6.5
CHD	2.6	1.5	7.0
High cholesterol	2.3	1.5	0.8

follow-up of women aged 40 to 64 in the American Cancer Society study who intentionally lost weight found a significant reduction in all-cause mortality of 20% to 25%.[24]

Weight loss affects a number of risk factors. The data on participants in the Swedish Obesity Study show the degree of weight loss for individual risk factors. Changes in blood pressure and triglycerides are very responsive to weight loss, decreasing after a 5% to 10% weight loss. HDL cholesterol increases with a similar weight-related change. Total cholesterol, on the other hand, does not show a sustained effect until weight loss exceeds 20%. For most comorbidities, however, a 10% weight loss is sufficient to see significant improvement in risk factors.[23,25]

Morbidity Associated With Obesity and Increased Central Fat
Overall Morbidity

Table 2 shows the relative risks for a variety of conditions, including hypertension, diabetes mellitus, and hy-

	Women	
White	African American	Mexican American
15.7	20.0	4.6
10.4	3.5	3.1
7.8	9.8	4.4
3.3	2.8	5.4
1.1	1 7	0.8

percholesterolemia, among overweight individuals. Overweight obviously greatly affects several diseases, but is only one of several factors. Sjostrom et al evaluated the 2-year incidence rate of new cases of disease in the overweight control group of the Swedish Obesity Study. In this population, the incidence of new cases of hypertension was 15%, 7.8% for new cases of diabetes, 5.8% for hyperinsulinemia, 27.8% for hypertriglyceridemia, and 15.9% for increased HDL cholesterol in this follow-up of untreated patients with a BMI averaging 38 kg/m^2 [23]

The risk of developing diabetes, hypertension, gallbladder disease, and coronary artery disease differs by ethnic group and by gender within ethnic group (Table 3). This is particularly evident for BMI >40 kg/m^2, but is also present at BMI between 30 and 40 kg/m^2.[26] In white women, the risk of noninsulin-dependent diabetes mellitus (NIDDM) was greater than the risk of hypertension, which in turn was greater than the risk of gallbladder disease. Although the risk of diabetes was also high in white

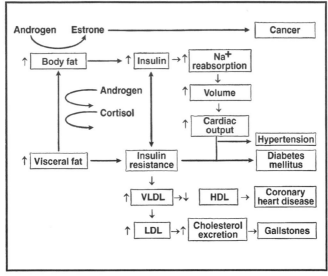

Figure 9: Factors influencing accumulation of visceral fat and its effect on mortality (copyright 1995, George A. Bray).

men, the risk of gallbladder disease exceeded that of hypertension, as opposed to white women. In African-American and Mexican-American men, the risk of hypertension was higher than that of diabetes. In African-American women, the risks of diabetes and gallbladder disease were higher whereas, in Mexican-American women, risks of coronary heart disease, diabetes, and gallbladder disease were similar, and the odds ratio was less than in corresponding African-American or white women. These ethnic and gender differences undoubtedly reflect the interaction of genetic and environmental factors.

Pathophysiology From Excess Fat

Each disease whose risk is increased by overweight can be classified into one of two pathophysiologic cat-

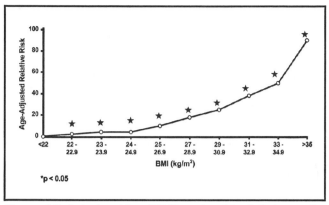

Figure 10: Relationship of BMI to the risk of diabetes. For each higher BMI above 22 kg/m², the incidence of diabetes mellitus further increased.[28]

egories. The first category is risks that result from the metabolic changes associated with excess fat. These include diabetes mellitus, gallbladder disease, hypertension, cardiovascular disease, and some forms of cancer associated with overweight. The second group of disabilities arises from the increased mass of fat itself. These include osteoarthritis, sleep apnea, and the stigma of obesity.

The fat cell can be viewed as a type of endocrine organ (Chapter 2). After the identification of adipsin or complement D in the fat cell, a number of other secretory peptides were found (Chapter 2). Leptin clearly is most important, and cements the role of the adipocyte as an endocrine cell and fat as an endocrine organ. From the pathophysiologic perspective, however, the release of free fatty acids is most important.

Fat distribution is important in the response to the endocrine products of the fat cell. The accumulation of body fat in visceral fat cells is modulated by a number of factors, some of which are presented schematically

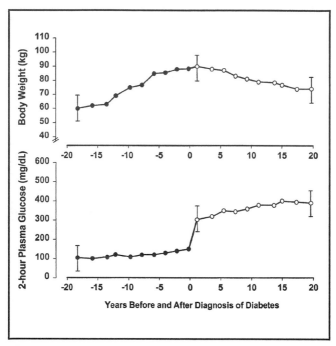

Figure 11: *Relationship of weight gain to development of diabetes in the Pima Indians.[28]*

in Figure 9. Androgens and estrogen produced by the gonads and adrenals, as well as peripheral conversion of Δ^4-androstenedione to estrone in fat cells, are pivotal in body fat distribution. Male or android fat distribution, and female or gynoid fat distribution, develop during adolescence. The increasing accumulation of visceral fat in adult life is related to gender, but the effects of cortisol, decreasing growth hormone, and changing testosterone levels are important in age-related fat accumulation. Increased visceral fat enhances the degree of insulin resistance associated with obesity and hyperinsulinemia. Together, hyperinsulinemia and insulin resistance enhance the risk of the comorbidities described below.

Diabetes Mellitus

Type II, or noninsulin-dependent diabetes mellitus (NIDDM), is strongly associated with overweight in both genders in all ethnic groups.[1] The risk of NIDDM increases with the degree and duration of overweight, and with a more central distribution of body fat. The relationship between increasing BMI and the risk of diabetes in the Health Professionals Study is shown in Figure 10.[27] The risk of diabetes was lowest in individuals with a BMI below 24 kg/m². As BMI increased, the relative risk increased such that at a BMI of 35 kg/m², the relative risk increased 40-fold, or 4,000%. A similar strong curvilinear relationship was observed in women in the Nurses' Health Study. The lowest risk in women was associated with a BMI below 22 kg/m², slightly lower than in the Health Professionals Study. At a BMI above 35 kg/m², the age-adjusted relative risk for diabetes in nurses increased to 60.9, or more than 6,000%.[28]

Weight gain also increases the risk of diabetes. More than 80% of NIDDM cases can be attributed to overweight. Of the 11.7 million cases of diabetes, overweight may account for two thirds of diabetic deaths. Using the BMI at age 18, a 20-kg weight gain increased the risk for diabetes 15-fold, whereas a weight reduction of 20 kg reduced the risk to almost zero. In the Health Professionals Study, weight gain was also associated with an increasing risk of NIDDM, whereas a 3-kg weight loss was associated with a reduction in relative risk.[27]

Weight gain appears to precede the onset of diabetes. Among the Pima Indians, body weight steadily and slowly increased by 30 kg (from 60 kg to 90 kg) in the years preceding the diagnosis of diabetes (Figure 11).[29] After the diagnosis of diabetes, body weight slightly decreased. In the Health Professionals Study, relative risk

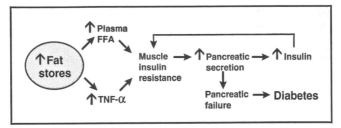

Figure 12: Pathophysiology of diabetes in overweight individuals.

of developing diabetes increased with weight gain, as well as with increased BMI.[28] In long-term follow-up studies, the duration of overweight and the change in plasma glucose during an oral glucose tolerance test also were strongly related. When overweight was present for less than 10 years, plasma glucose was not increased. With longer durations, of up to 45 years, a nearly linear increase in plasma glucose occurred after an oral glucose tolerance test. Risk of diabetes is increased in hypertensive individuals treated with diuretics or b-blocking drugs, and this risk was increased in the overweight.

In the Swedish Obesity Study, Sjostrom et al observed that diabetes was present in 13% to 16% of obese subjects at baseline.[23] Of those who underwent gastric bypass and subsequently lost weight, 69% who initially had diabetes were cured, and only 0.5% of those who did not have diabetes at baseline developed it. In contrast, in the obese control group that lost no weight, the cure rate was low, 16%, and the incidence of new cases of diabetes was 7.8%.

Weight loss or moderating weight gain over years reduces the risk of developing diabetes. This is most clearly shown in the Health Professionals Study, in which relative risk declined by nearly 50% with a weight loss of 5 to 11 kg. Type II diabetes was almost nonexistent with a weight loss of more than 20 kg or a BMI below 20 kg/m^2.[28]

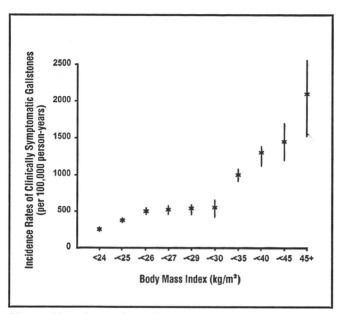

Figure 13: *Relationship of BMI to the development of gallbladder disease.*[30]

A pathophysiologic model for diabetes is shown in Figure 12. Both increased insulin secretion and insulin resistance are part of obesity. The relationship of insulin secretion to BMI already has been noted. Greater BMI correlates with greater insulin secretion. Obesity develops in more than 50% of nonhuman primates as they age. Nearly half of these obese animals subsequently develop diabetes. The time course for the development of obesity in nonhuman primates, like in the Pima Indians, is spread over a number of years. After the animals gain weight, the next demonstrable effects are impaired glucose removal and increased insulin resistance as measured by impaired glucose clearance with an euglycemic hyperinsulinemic clamp. The hyperinsulinemia in turn increases hepatic VLDL triglyceride synthesis and se-

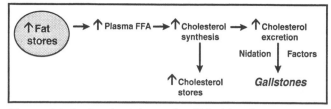

Figure 14: Pathophysiology of gallbladder disease in overweight individuals.

cretion, increases plasminogen activator inhibitor-1 (PAI-1) synthesis, increases sympathetic nervous system activity, and increases renal sodium reabsorption.

Insulin resistance decreases the glut-4 glucose transporter in adipose tissue, and decreases glucokinase activity in the liver. The promoter region of the genes for these two enzymes has an insulin-response element and a peroxisome-proliferater activator receptor-γ (PPAR-γ) response element. Insulin resistance may reflect a reduction in the occupancy of the PPAR-γ response element, with reduced transcription of these two components of glucose metabolism. A factor from adipose tissue, such as leptin or TNF-α, or some undescribed peptide or rexinoid, might impair PPAR-γ activation and thus diminish the response to insulin and lower glut-4 and glucokinase, producing insulin resistance. Diabetes would then develop in individuals in whom pancreatic β-cell production was unable to provide sufficient insulin (Figure 12).

Gallbladder Disease

Cholelithiasis is the primary hepatobiliary pathology associated with overweight.[4] The old clinical adage 'fat, female, fertile, and forty' describes the epidemiologic factors often involved in the development of gallbladder disease. This is admirably demonstrated in the Nurses' Health Study[30] (Figure 13). When BMI was below

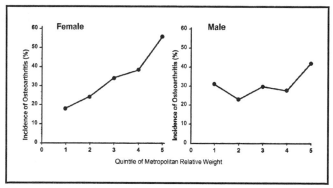

Figure 15: *Incidence of osteoarthritis in relation to BMI.*[30]

24 kg/m^2, the incidence of clinically symptomatic gall-stones was approximately 250 per 100,000 person-years of follow-up. Incidence gradually increased with increased BMI (to 30 kg/m^2) and increased very steeply when BMI exceeded 30 kg/m^2. This confirms published work by many other researchers.

Part of the explanation for the increased risk of gall-stones is the increased cholesterol turnover related to total body fat.[4] Cholesterol production is linearly related to body fat; approximately 20 mg of additional cholesterol is synthesized for each kilogram of extra body fat. Thus, a 10-kg increase in body fat leads to the daily synthesis of as much cholesterol as is contained in the yolk of one egg. The increased cholesterol is in turn excreted in the bile. High cholesterol concentrations relative to bile acids and phospholipids in bile increase the likelihood of precipitation of cholesterol gallstones in the gallbladder. Additional factors, such as nidation conditions, also are involved in whether gallstones form[4] (Figure 14).

During weight loss, the likelihood of gallstones increases because the flux of cholesterol is increased through the biliary system. Diets with moderate levels

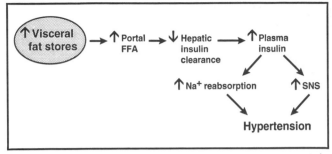

Figure 16: *Pathophysiology of hypertension in overweight individuals.*

of fat that trigger gallbladder contraction and thus empty the cholesterol content may reduce this risk. Similarly, the use of bile acids, such as ursodeoxycholic acid, may be advisable if the risk of gallstone formation is thought to be increased.

The second GI feature altered in obesity is the quantity of fat in the liver.[4] Increased steatosis is characteristic of the livers of overweight people, and may reflect increased VLDL production associated with hyperinsulinemia. The accumulation of lipid in the liver suggests that the secretion of VLDL in response to hyperinsulinemia is inadequate to keep up with the high rate of triglyceride turnover.

Bones, Joints, Muscles, Connective Tissue, and Skin

Osteoarthritis is significantly increased in overweight individuals. The osteoarthritis that develops in the knees and ankles may be directly related to the trauma associated with the degree of excess body weight (Figure 15).[31] However, the increased osteoarthritis in other nonweight-bearing joints suggests that some components of the overweight syndrome alter cartilage and bone metabolism, independent of weight bearing. Increased osteoarthritis

Table 4: Comparison of Cardiac Structural and Hemodynamic Alterations in Patients With Obesity Alone, Systemic Hypertension Alone, and Combined Obesity and Hypertension[32]

Variable	Obesity Alone	Hypertension Alone	Obesity and Hypertension
Heart rate	N	N	N
Blood pressure	N	↑	↑
Stroke volume	↑	N	↑
Cardiac output	↑	N	↑
Systemic vascular resistance	↓	↑	N or ↑
LV volume	↑	N	↑
LV wall stress	N or ↑	N or ↑	↑
LV hypertrophy	Eccentric	Concentric	Hybrid
LV diastolic dysfunction	Usually present	Usually present	Usually present
LV systolic dysfunction	Occasionally present	Usually absent	Occasionally present
LV failure	Occasionally present	Occasionally present	Common
RV hypertrophy	Occasionally present	Usually absent	Occasionally present
RV enlargement	Occasionally present	Usually absent	Occasionally present
RV failure	Occasionally present	Usually absent	Occasionally present

accounts for a significant component of the cost of over-weight (Table 1).

Several skin changes are associated with excess weight. Stretch marks, or striae, are common and reflect the pressures on the skin from expanding lobular deposits of fat. Acanthosis nigricans with deepening pigmentation in the folds of the neck, knuckles and extensor surfaces occurs in many overweight individuals, but is not associated with increased risk of malignancy. Hirsutism in women may reflect the altered reproductive status in these individuals.

Hypertension

Blood pressure often is increased in overweight individuals[5] (Figure 16). In the Swedish Obesity Study, hypertension was present at baseline in 44% to 51% of subjects. One estimate suggests that control of overweight would eliminate 48% of the hypertension in whites and 28% in blacks. For each decline of 1 mm Hg in diastolic blood pressure, the risk of myocardial infarction decreases an estimated 2% to 3%.

Overweight and hypertension interact with cardiac function. Hypertension in normal-weight people produces concentric hypertrophy of the heart with thickening of the ventricular walls. In overweight individuals, eccentric dilatation occurs. Increased preload and stroke work are associated with hypertension. The combination of overweight and hypertension leads to thickening of the ventricular wall and larger heart volume, and thus to a greater likelihood of cardiac failure. Table 4 summarizes the changes in overweight with and without hypertension.[32]

The hypertension of overweight people appears strongly related to altered sympathetic activity (Figure 16). During insulin infusion, overweight subjects have a much greater increase in muscle sympathetic nerve firing rate than do normal-weight subjects, but the altered

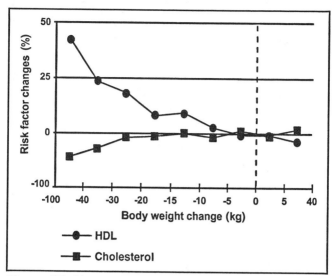

Figure 17: Changes in total cholesterol and HDL cholesterol with weight loss.[23]

activity is associated with a lesser change in the vascular resistance of calf muscles.

Hypertension is strongly associated with type II diabetes, impaired glucose tolerance, hypertriglyceridemia, and hypercholesterolemia. This association or symptom cluster is the *insulin resistance syndrome*, the *metabolic syndrome*, or *syndrome X*. In 2,930 subjects, these conditions individually were associated with a 1.5% incidence of hypertension, compared with a rate of 11.1% for hypertension when the other factors also were present.[33] Hyperinsulinemia in overweight and in hypertensive patients suggests insulin resistance. An analysis of the factors that predict blood pressure and changes in peripheral vascular resistance in response to body weight showed that a key determinant of the weight-induced increases in blood pressure was a disproportionate increase in cardiac output that could not be fully ac-

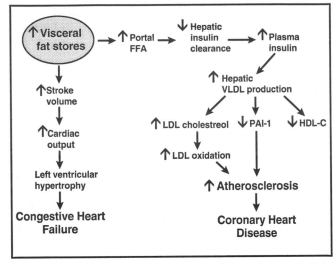

Figure 18: Pathophysiology of heart disease in overweight individuals.

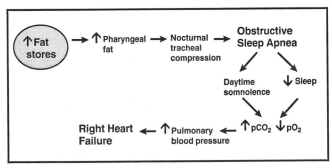

Figure 19: Pathophysiology of sleep apnea in overweight individuals.

counted for by the hemodynamic contribution of new tissue. This hemodynamic change may be attributable to a disproportionate increase in cardiac output related to an increase in sympathetic activity.

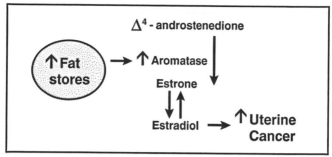

Figure 20: *Pathophysiology of uterine cancer in overweight women.*

In experimental studies in which animals are force-fed to produce obesity, the response to chronic insulin infusion depends on the species. In dogs made obese by a high-fat diet, hyperinsulinemia had no increased pressor effect. In rats, on the other hand, 7 days of insulin infusion produced a sustained increase in arterial blood pressure. The key is whether overweight human beings respond to insulin more like the rat or the dog. This question remains to be resolved.

Heart Disease

Data from the Nurses' Health Study indicate that the risk for U.S. women developing coronary artery disease is increased 3.3-fold with a BMI >29 kg/m², compared with women with a BMI <21 kg/m².[14] A BMI 27 to <29 kg/m² increases the relative risk to 1.8 (Figure 3). Weight gain also strongly affects this risk at any initial BMI.[20] That is, at all levels of initial BMI, weight gain was associated with a graded increase in risk of heart disease. This was particularly evident in the highest quintile in which weight gain was more than 20 kg.

Dyslipidemia may be important in the relationship of BMI to increased risk of heart disease.[2] A positive correlation between BMI and triglyceride has been repeat-

Table 5: Common Hormonal Abnormalities Associated With Obesity

- Increased cortisol production
- Insulin resistance
- Decreased sex hormone-binding globulin (SHBG) in women
- Decreased progesterone levels in women
- Decreased testosterone levels in men
- Decreased growth hormone production

edly demonstrated. However, the inverse relationship between HDL cholesterol and BMI may be more important because a low HDL cholesterol carries a greater relative risk than do elevated triglycerides. Central fat distribution also is important in lipid abnormalities. Waist circumference alone accounted for as much as or more of the variance in triglycerides and HDL cholesterol than either WHR or sagittal diameter. A positive correlation for central fat and triglyceride and the inverse relationship for HDL cholesterol is evident for all measures. A detailed analysis showed that waist circumference better correlated with lipids than did sagittal diameter, and both were better than WHR. Like most other risk factors, weight loss lowers cholesterol slightly and raises HDL cholesterol (Figure 17).

Increased body weight is associated with a number of cardiovascular abnormalities.[32] Cardiac weight increases with increasing body weight, suggesting increased cardiac work. Heart weight as a percentage of body weight is lower than in a normal-weight control group. The increased cardiac work associated with overweight may

Table 6: Estimated Effect of Overweight in Adolescence on Subsequent Social and Economic Characteristics and Self-Esteem Among Women[36]

Variable	Observed Value		P Value
	Overweight (N=195)	Nonoverweight (N=4,943)	
Married (n=4,922)	28%	56%	<0.001
Household income (n=4,286)	$18,372	$30,586	<0.001
Income below poverty level[a] (n=4,286)	32%	13%	<0.001
Education (n=4,881)	12.1 years	13.1 years	0.009
Completed college (n=4,881)	9%	21%	0.21
Self-esteem scale in 1987 (n=5,138)	32.4	33.6	0.38

[a]Household poverty defined according to federal poverty guidelines.

produce cardiomyopathy and heart failure. Weight loss decreases heart weight; this decrease was linearly related to the degree of weight loss in both men and women.

Echocardiographic study of left ventricular midwall function showed that obese individuals compensated by using cardiac reserve, especially in the presence of hypertension. Interestingly, heart rate was well within normal. A pathophysiologic diagram for the observed changes is shown in Figure 18. The diagram has two parts. Portal fatty acids increase insulin, which increases hepatic triglyceride production. This, and the changes in fat cell size, change cholesterol production as well as the rate of PAI-1 production. The net effects are the changes of atherosclerosis. The second effect of enlargement of fat cells is an increased capillary bed and blood flow. This can lead to congestive heart failure.

Central fat distribution is associated with small dense low-density lipoproteins (LDL) as opposed to the large fluffy LDL.[2] For a similar level of cholesterol, the risk of coronary heart disease (CHD) is significantly higher in individuals with small dense LDL than with large fluffy LDL. Because each LDL particle has a single molecule of apo B protein, the concentration of apo B can be used to estimate the number of LDL particles. Despres et al demonstrated that the level of apo B is a strong predictor of the risk for CHD.[2] Based on a study of French Canadians, the researchers proposed that estimating apo B, the levels of fasting insulin, the concentration of triglyceride, the concentration of HDL cholesterol, and waist circumference could help identify individuals at high risk for the metabolic syndrome (see Chapter 5).

Respiratory System

Alterations in pulmonary function have been described in overweight subjects, but subjects were free of other potential chronic pulmonary diseases in only a few studies. In studies of individuals without underlying pulmonary disease, only major degrees of increased body weight significantly affected pulmonary function.

The chief effect is a decrease in residual lung volume associated with increased abdominal pressure on the diaphragm.[34] Fat distribution, independent of total fat, also influences ventilatory capacity in men, possibly through effects of visceral fat level.

In contrast to the relatively benign effects of excess weight on respiratory function, the overweight associated with sleep apnea can be severe.[34] A pathophysiologic sequence is presented in Figure 19. Overweight subjects with obstructive sleep apnea show a number of significant differences from overweight subjects without sleep apnea. Sleep apnea was considerably more common in men than women and, as a group, subjects were significantly taller than individuals without sleep apnea. People with sleep apnea have an increased snoring index and increased maximal nocturnal sound intensity. Nocturnal oxygen saturation also was significantly reduced. One interesting hypothesis is that the increased neck circumference and fat deposits in the pharyngeal area may lead to the obstructive sleep apnea of obesity.

Cancer

Certain forms of cancer are significantly increased in overweight individuals (Figure 3).[12] Males face increased risk for neoplasms of the colon, rectum, and prostate. In women, cancers of the reproductive system and gallbladder are more common. One explanation for the increased risk of endometrial cancer in overweight women is the increased production of estrogens by adipose tissue stromal cells (Figure 20). This increased production is related to the degree of excess body fat that accounts for a major source of estrogen production in postmenopausal women. Breast cancer is not only related to total body fat, but also may have a more important relationship to central body fat.[35] The increased visceral fat measured by computed tomography shows an important relationship to the risk of breast cancer.

Endocrine Changes

A variety of endocrine changes are associated with overweight (Table 5). The changes in the reproductive system are among the most important. Irregular menses and frequent anovular cycles are common, and the rate of fertility may be reduced. Some reports describe increased risks of toxemia. Hypertension and cesarean section may be more frequent.

Psychosocial Function

Overweight is stigmatized,[36] that is, overweight individuals are exposed to the consequences of public disapproval of their fatness. This stigma occurs in education, employment, and health care, and elsewhere (Table 6). Psychosocial consequences are revealed by examining education, marital status, and income level in adolescents who were overweight into adult life. These effects were more evident in females than in males.

References

1.　Albu J, Pi-Sunyer FX: Obesity and diabetes. In: Bray GA, Bouchard C, James WP, eds. *Handbook of Obesity.* New York, Marcel Dekker, 1997, pp 697-707.

2.　Despres JP, Krauss RM: Obesity and lipoprotein metabolism. In: Bray GA, Bouchard C, James WP, eds. *Handbook of Obesity.* New York, Marcel Dekker, 1997, pp 651-675.

3.　Kissebah AH, Krakower GR: Regional adiposity and morbidity. *Physiol Rev* 1994;74:761-811.

4.　Ko CW, Lee SP: Obesity and gallbladder disease. In: Bray GA, Bouchard C, James WP, eds. *Handbook of Obesity.* New York, Marcel Dekker, 1997, pp 709-724.

5.　Rocchini AP: Obesity and blood pressure regulation. In: Bray GA, Bouchard C, James WP, eds. *Handbook of Obesity.* New York, Marcel Dekker, 1997, pp 677-695.

6.   Sjostrom LV: Morbidity of severely obese subjects. *Am J Clin Nutr* 1992;55:508S-515S.

7.   Sjostrom LV: Mortality of severely obese subjects. *Am J Clin Nutr* 1992;55:516S-523S.

8.   Wolf AM, Colditz GA: Current estimates of the economic cost of obesity in the United States. *Obes Res* 1998;6:97-106.

9.   Caan B, Quesenberry CP Jr, Jacobson A: Increase in health care costs associated with obesity. *Obes Res* 1997;5:5S.

10.   Sjostrom L, Larsson B, Backman L, et al: Swedish obese subjects (SOS). Recruitment for an intervention study and a selected description of the obese state. *Int J Obes Relat Metab Disord* 1992;16:465-479.

11.   Society of Actuaries: *Build Study of 1979.* Chicago, Society of Actuaries/Association of Life Insurance Medical Directors of America, 1980.

12.   Lew EA: Mortality and weight: insured lives and the American Cancer Society studies. *Ann Intern Med* 1985;103:1024-1029.

13.   Waaler HT: Height, weight and mortality. The Norwegian experience. *Acta Med Scand Suppl* 1984;679:1-56.

14.   Manson JE, Willett WC, Stampfer MJ, et al: Body weight and mortality among women. *N Engl J Med* 1995;333:677-685.

15.   Manson JE, Stampfer MJ, Hennekens CH, et al: Body weight and longevity. A reassessment. *JAMA* 1987;257:353-358.

16.   Sonne-Holm S, Sorensen TI, Christensen U: Risk of early death in extremely overweight young men. *Br Med J (Clin Res Ed)* 1983;287:795-797.

17.   Bray GA: Coherent preventive and management strategies for obesity. In: Chadwick DJ, Cardew G, eds. *The Origins and Consequences of Obesity.* Ciba Foundation Symposium 201. London, John Wiley, 1996, pp 228-246.

18.   McGinnis JM, Foege WH: Actual causes of death in the United States. *JAMA* 1993;270:2207-2212.

19.   Lapidus L, Bengtsson C, Larsson B. et al: Distribution of adipose tissue and risk of cardiovascular disease and death: a 12 year follow up of participants in the population study of women in Gothenburg, Sweden. *Br Med J (Clin Res Ed)* 1984;289:1257-1261.

20.   Willett WC, Manson JE, Stampfer MJ, et al: Weight, weight change, and coronary heart disease in women. Risk within the 'normal' weight range. *JAMA* 1995;273:461-465.

21. Blair SN, Kohl HW 3d, Paffenbarger RS Jr, et al: Physical fitness and all-cause mortality. A prospective study of healthy men and women. *JAMA* 1989;262:2395-2401.

22. World Health Organization: *Obesity: Preventing and Managing the Global Epidemic.* Report of a WHO Consultation on Obesity, Geneva, June 1997.

23. Sjostrom CD, Lissner L, Sjostrom L: Relationships between changes in body composition and changes in cardiovascular risk factors: the SOS Intervention Study. Swedish Obese Subjects. *Obes Res* 1997;5:519-530.

24. Williamson DF, Pamuk E, Thun M, et al: Prospective study of intentional weight loss and mortality in never-smoking overweight US white women aged 40-64 years. *Am J Epidemiol* 1995;141:1128-1141.

25. Institute of Medicine (IOM). In: Thomas PR, ed. *Weighing the Options: Criteria for Evaluating Weight-Management Programs.* Washington, DC, National Academy Press, 1995.

26. Must A, Spadano J, Dietz WH: Prevalence of obesity-related morbidity in relation to adult overweight in the United States. *Obes Res* 5:27S.

27. Chan JM, Rimm EB, Colditz GA, et al: Obesity, fat distribution, and weight gain as risk factors for clinical diabetes in men. *Diabetes Care* 1994;17:961-969.

28. Colditz GA, Willett WC, Rotnitzky A, et al: Weight gain as a risk factor for clinical diabetes mellitus in women. *Ann Intern Med* 1995;122:481-486.

29. Ravussin E: Energy metabolism in obesity. Studies in the Pima Indians. *Diabetes Care* 1993;16:232-238.

30. Stampfer MJ, Maclure KM, Colditz GA, et al: Risk of symptomatic gallstones in women with severe obesity. *Am J Clin Nutr* 1992;55:652-658.

31. Felson DT, Anderson JJ, Naimark A, et al: Obesity and knee osteoarthritis. The Framingham Study. *Ann Intern Med* 1988;109:18-24.

32. Alpert MA, Hashimi MW: Obesity and the heart. *Am J Med Sci* 1993;306:117-123.

33. Ferrannini E, Haffner SM, Mitchell BD, et al: Hyperinsulinaemia: the key feature of a cardiovascular and metabolic syndrome. *Diabetologia* 1991;34:416-422.

34.   Strohl KP, Strobel RJ, Parisi RA: Obesity and pulmonary function. In: Bray GA, Bouchard C, James WP, eds. *Handbook of Obesity*. New York, Marcel Dekker, 1997, pp 725-739.

35.   Schapira DV, Clark RA, Wolff PA, et al: Visceral obesity and breast cancer risk. *Cancer* 1994;74:632-639.

36.   Gortmaker SL, Must A, Perrin JM, et al: Social and economic consequences of overweight in adolescence and young adulthood. *N Engl J Med* 1993;329:1008-1012.

Chapter 4

Clinical Classification and Natural History of Overweight

"All disease entities are abstract concepts created by the human mind."

— Faber, 1923

*"They are sick that surfeit with too much
As they that starve with nothing."*

— Shakespeare
The Merchant of Venice
Act I, Scene 1

This chapter examines clinical features of overweight. The first section presents two ways to classify overweight individuals: anatomic and etiologic. The second section addresses the natural history of overweight and the factors that contribute to the onset of overweight through the life span.

Clinical Classification

Anatomic Characteristics of Adipose Tissue and Fat Distribution

An anatomic classification of obesity can be based on the number of adipocytes, on the regional distribution of body fat, or on the characteristics of localized fat deposits.[1,2]

Number of Fat Cells

The number of fat cells can be estimated from the total amount of body fat and the average size of a fat cell. Because fat cells differ in size by body region, a reliable estimate of the total number of fat cells should be based on the average fat cell size from more than one location. In adults, the upper limits of total normal fat cells range from 40×10^9 to 60×10^9. The number of fat cells increases most rapidly during late childhood and puberty, but may increase even in adult life. The number of fat cells can increase 3- to 5-fold when obesity occurs in childhood or adolescence.

Hypercellular obesity (ie, obesity with an increased number of fat cells) shows varying degrees of enlargement of fat cells. This type of obesity usually begins in early or middle childhood, but may also occur in adult life. An increased number of fat cells usually accompanies a body mass index (BMI) above 40 kg/m².

Hypertrophic obesity (ie, obesity with enlarged fat cells but not an increased number of fat cells) tends to correlate with an android or truncal fat distribution, and often is associated with metabolic disorders such as glucose intolerance, dyslipidemia, hypertension, and coronary artery disease.

Fat Distribution

Fat distribution can be estimated by a variety of techniques (Chapter 1). The ratio of waist circumference to hip circumference (WHR) was used in the pioneering studies that brought scientific recognition in the 1980s to the relationship of central fat to disease, a concept originally suggested by Vague. The subscapular skinfold also has been valuable in estimating central fat in epidemiologic studies. A more sophisticated technique to evaluate skinfolds uses principal component analysis of skinfolds at several body sites. This analysis groups the skinfolds that are best correlated, and estimates total fat, central fat, and peripheral fat. Reliable estimates of visceral fat, however, can only be made by computed tomography (CT) or magnetic resonance imaging (MRI). Waist circumference alone and WHR are used in Chapter 5 as one criterion for evaluating health risk from obesity.

Localized Deposits of Fat and Lipodystrophy

Localized fat accumulations include single lipomas, multiple lipomas, liposarcomas, and lipodystrophy.[2] Lipomas vary in size from 1 cm to more than 15 cm. They can occur in any body region, and represent encapsulated accumulations of fat. Multiple lipomatosis is an inherited disease transmitted as an autosomal dominant trait. Von Recklinghausen's syndrome, Maffucci's syndrome, and Madelung's deformity are lipomatous syndromes.

Liposarcomas are relatively rare, representing less than 1% of lipomas. They tend to affect the lower extremities and consist of 4 types: well-differentiated myxoid; poorly differentiated myxoid; round cell or adenoid; and mixed.[2]

Weber-Christian disease and Dercum's disease are idiopathic accumulations of fat. Dercum's disease, also called adiposis dolorosa, is named after the painful nodules in the subcutaneous fat of middle-aged women. Weber-Christian disease, on the other hand, is a relapsing febrile disease occurring in younger women. All of these forms of localized fat deposits are relatively rare.[2]

Lipodystrophy is a loss of body fat in one or more body regions. Total lipodystrophy is a familial disease with absent subcutaneous fat. Partial lipodystrophy usually is acquired, and can affect the upper or lower body. Total fat metabolism appears accelerated in the affected regions.

Etiologic Classification

Neuroendocrine Obesity

A variety of neuroendocrine disorders may be associated with the development of obesity.

Hypothalamic obesity. Hypothalamic obesity is rare in humans. It can be regularly produced in animals by injuring the ventromedial or paraventricular region of the hypothalamus or the amygdala (Chapter 2).[3] These brain regions are responsible for integrating metabolic

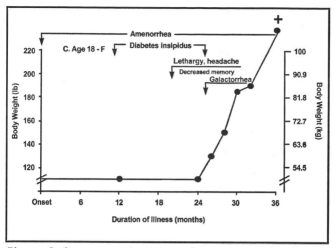

Figure 1: *Symptomatic course of a patient with tuberculomas and hypothalamic obesity. Numerous symptoms developed in the first 2 years, followed by rapid weight gain in the third year.*

information on nutrient stores with afferent sensory information on food availability. When the ventromedial hypothalamus is damaged, hyperphagia develops and obesity follows.

Hypothalamic obesity in humans may be caused by trauma, tumor, inflammatory disease, surgery in the posterior fossa, or increased intracranial pressure.[4] The symptoms usually present in one of three patterns: (1) headache, vomiting, and diminished vision; (2) impaired endocrine function affecting the reproductive system with amenorrhea or impotence, diabetes insipidus, and thyroid or adrenal insufficiency; or (3) neurologic and physiologic derangements, including convulsions, coma, somnolence, and hypothermia or hyperthermia (Table 1). One clinical presentation is shown in Figure 1. Weight gain occurred in the third year after the appearance of several endocrine and hypothalamic changes. The patient died

Table 1: Hypothalamic Obesity

Hypothalamic Lesions
- tumors
- inflammation
- trauma

Endocrine Disturbances
- amenorrhea/impotence
- impaired growth
- diabetes insipidus
- thyroid/adrenal insufficiency

Intracranial Pressure
- papilledema
- vomiting

Neurologic Disturbances
- thirst
- somnolence

with multiple tuberculomas in the hypothalamus despite triple-antibiotic therapy.

Cushing's syndrome. A common clinical feature in patients with Cushing's syndrome is progressive central obesity, usually involving the face, neck (leading to a buffalo hump and obscuring the clavicles), trunk, abdomen and, internally, the mesentery and mediastinum.[5] The extremities usually are spared and often are wasted (Table 2).

In contrast to adults, nearly all children with Cushing's syndrome have generalized obesity accompanied by a decrease in linear growth. As a result, any child whose weight rises and whose stature remains static when compared with age-matched normally growing children should be evaluated for Cushing's syndrome. The differential diagnosis of obesity and Cushing's disease is clinically important

Table 2: Cushing's Syndrome

- Central obesity
- Hypertension
- Plethoric facies
- Amenorrhea
- Virilism
- Edema of lower extremities
- Hemorrhagic features

Table 3: Polycystic Ovary Syndrome

- Oligomenorrhea/amenorrhea
- Hirsutism
- Polycystic ovaries
- Increased LH/FSH
- Increased testosterone/decreased SHBG
- Insulin resistance
- Normal IGF-1
- Decreased IGF-1 binding protein

for therapeutic decisions. Three screening tests can be used to select patients for a final dexamethasone-corticotropin releasing hormone (CRH) test: (1) 24-hour urinary free cortisol (normal <150 nmol/24 h); (2) cortisol production rate (normal <80 nmol/kg/24 h); and (3) overnight dexamethasone suppression test (0.5 mg dexamethasone at midnight—a.m. plasma cortisol <75 nmol/L). Any patient who tests abnormal should receive dexamethasone 0.5 mg every 6 h for 2 days, followed by 100 µg of CRH intravenously. A normal value for this dexamethasone-CRH test is cortisol <38 nmol/L 15 minutes after CRH.[6]

Hypothyroidism. Patients with hypothyroidism frequently gain weight because of a generalized slowing of metabolic activity. Some of this gain is fat. However, the weight gain usually is modest, and marked obesity is uncommon. Hypothyroidism is common, particularly in older women. In this group, a thyroid-stimulating hormone (TSH) test (Chapter 5) is valuable.

Polycystic ovary syndrome. More than 50% of women with polycystic ovary syndrome (PCOS) are obese.[7] The cardinal features of this syndrome are oligomenorrhea, hirsutism, and polycystic ovaries. Although obesity is not always present, it occurs more often than not. Insulin resistance is present in both normal and overweight patients. Luteinizing hormone (LH) usually is increased, and ovarian overproduction of testosterone, probably through ovarian stimulation by insulin-like growth factor-1 (IGF-1), is a main source of testosterone. The factors responsible for this association are not understood (Table 3).

Growth hormone. Lean body mass is decreased and fat mass is increased in adults who are deficient in growth hormone, compared with those who have normal growth hormone secretion. Growth hormone replacement reduces body and visceral fat.[8] Acromegaly produces the opposite effects with reduced body fat and particularly visceral fat. Treatment of acromegaly, which lowers growth hormone, increases body fat and visceral fat. The gradual decline in growth hormone with age may be one reason for the increase in visceral fat with age.

Drug-Induced Weight Gain

Several drugs can cause weight gain, including a variety of psychoactive agents and hormones (Table 4). The degree of weight gain is generally not sufficient to cause true obesity, except occasionally in patients treated with high-dose corticosteroids. Antipsychotics (phenothiazines and butyrophenones) often cause weight gain. One study found that men hospitalized for mental illness, many of whom were treated with phenothiazines, gained an aver-

Table 4: Drugs That Increase Body Weight

Antipsychotics (Phenothiazines and Butyrophenones):
chlorpromazine, thioridazine, trifluoperazine, mesoridazine, promazine, mepazine, perphenazine, prochlorperazine, haloperidol, loxapine

Antidepressants:
amitriptyline, imipramine, doxepin, phenelzine, amoxapine, desipramine, trazodone, tranylcypromine, lithium

Antiepileptics:
valproate, carbamazepine

Steroids:
glucocorticoids, megestrol acetate, estrogen

Adrenergic Antagonists:
α_1-antagonists, β_2-antagonists (weak)

Serotonin Antagonists:
cyproheptadine

Antidiabetics:
insulin, sulfonylureas

age of 3.2 kg over a stay of 35 months. Phenothiazines were thought particularly important in this weight gain. Among other psychotropic drugs, the tricyclic antidepressant amitriptyline (Elavil®) is likely to cause weight gain and a carbohydrate preference. Lithium also has been implicated in weight gain. Valproate (Depakene®) is an antiepileptic drug that acts on the NMDA (GABA) receptor. It causes weight gain in more than 50% of patients. Glucocorticoids cause fat accumulation in particular areas, similar to that of Cushing's syndrome. These changes occur mostly in patients taking prednisone 10 mg/d or more. Megestrol acetate (Megace®) is a progestin used in women with breast cancer and in patients with AIDS to increase appetite and induce weight gain.[9] The increase in weight is fat. The serotonin antagonist cyproheptadine (Periactin®) is associated with weight gain. Insulin stimulates appetite, probably through hypoglycemia. Weight gain occurs in diabetic patients treated with insulin or with sulfonylureas, which enhance endogenous insulin release. In contrast, weight gain is not a problem with hypoglycemic agents that increase insulin action, such as metformin (Glucophage®) or troglitazone (Rezulin®). In one large study, the administration of chlorpropamide (Diabinese®), glyburide (DiaBeta®, Glynase®, Micronase®), or insulin was associated with a 3.5- to 4.8-kg weight gain at 6 years, compared with no change with metformin.[10] The effect of insulin was dose dependent. In the Diabetes Control and Complications Trial, the mean increase in weight in patients with insulin-dependent diabetes was 5.1 kg with intensive insulin therapy, and 2.4 kg with conventional insulin therapy.[11]

Cessation of Smoking

Weight gain is very common when people stop smoking. Researchers believe this is at least partly mediated by nicotine withdrawal. Weight gain of 1 to 2 kg in the first few weeks is often followed by an additional 2- to 3-kg weight gain over the next 4 to 6 months. Average weight gain is 4 to 5 kg, but can be much greater.[12] Researchers have estimated that smoking cessation increases the odds ratio of obesity 2.4-fold in men and 2.0-fold in women, compared with nonsmokers.

The effects of smoking and smoking cessation on body weight have also been evaluated by comparing identical twin pairs to eliminate genetic and certain environmental factors. Light, moderate, and heavy smokers were an average of 3.2, 2.4, and 4.0 kg lighter than nonsmokers. On the other hand, past smokers had a significantly higher incidence of obesity (27%) than their currently smoking siblings. Because of the substantial predictability of weight gain after smoking cessation, an exercise program and decreased caloric intake are recommended for all patients who plan to stop smoking.

Sedentary Lifestyle

A sedentary lifestyle lowers energy expenditure and promotes weight gain in both animals and humans. Restriction of physical activity in rats causes weight gain, and animals in zoos tend to be heavier than those in the wild. In an affluent society, energy-sparing devices in the workplace and at home reduce energy expenditure and may enhance the tendency to gain weight.

A number of additional observations illustrate the importance of decreased energy expenditure in the pathogenesis of weight gain. The highest frequency of overweight occurs in men in sedentary occupations. Estimates of energy intake and energy expenditure in Great Britain suggest that reduced energy expenditure is more important than increased food intake in causing obesity.[13] A study of middle-aged men in the Netherlands found that the decline in energy expenditure accounted for almost all weight gain.[14] According to the Surgeon General's Report on Physical Activity,[15] the percentage of adult Americans participating in physical activity decreases steadily with age, and reduced energy expenditure in adults and children predicts weight gain.

Diet

The amount of energy intake relative to energy expenditure is crucial in the development of obesity. However, diet composition also may be variably important in its pathogenesis. Dietary factors become important in a variety of settings.

Overeating. Voluntary overeating (repeated ingestion of energy exceeding daily energy needs) can increase body weight in normal-weight men and women. When these subjects stop overeating, they invariably lose the excess weight. The use of overeating to study the consequences of food ingestion has shown the importance of genetic factors in the pattern of weight gain and subsequent loss.[16]

Restrained eating. A pattern of conscious limitation of food intake is 'restrained' eating.[17] It is common in many, if not most, middle-age women of 'normal weight.' It also may account for the inverse relationship of body weight to social class; women of upper socioeconomic status often use restrained eating to maintain their weight. In a weight-loss clinic, higher restraint scores were associated with lower body weights.[18] Weight loss was associated with a significant increase in restraint, indicating that higher levels of conscious control maintain lower weight. Greater increases in restraint correlate with greater weight loss, but also with higher risk of 'lapse' or loss of control and overeating.

Japanese sumo wrestlers who eat large quantities of food twice a day for many years, and who have a very active training schedule, have low visceral fat relative to total weight. When their active career ends, however, the wrestlers tend to remain overweight and have a high probability of developing diabetes mellitus.

Frequency of eating. The relationship between the frequency of meals and the development of obesity is unsettled. Many anecdotal reports argue that overweight persons eat less often than normal-weight persons, but documentation is difficult. However, frequency of eating does change lipid and glucose metabolism. When normal subjects eat several small meals a day, serum cholesterol concentrations are lower than when they eat a few large meals a day. Similarly, mean blood glucose concentrations are lower when meals are frequent.[19] One explanation for the effects of frequent small meals compared with a few large meals could be the greater insulin secretion associated with larger meals.

Dietary fat intake. Epidemiologic data suggest that a high-fat diet is associated with obesity. The relative weight in several populations, for example, is directly related to the percentage of dietary fat.[20] A high-fat diet introduces palatable, often high-fat foods into the diet, with a corresponding increase in energy density (ie, lesser weight of food for the same number of calories). This makes overconsumption more likely. Differences in the storage capacity for various macronutrients also may be involved. Carbohydrate stores are limited by the capacity to store glycogen in liver and muscle, and they need to be replenished frequently. This contrasts with fat stores, which are more than 100 times the daily intake of fat. This difference in storage capacity makes eating carbohydrates a more important physiologic need that may lead to overeating when dietary carbohydrate is limited (Chapter 2) and carbohydrate oxidation cannot be sufficiently reduced.

Night-eating syndrome. The night-eating syndrome is the consumption of at least 25% (and usually more than 50%) of energy between the evening meal and the next morning. It is a common pattern of disturbed eating in the obese. It is related to sleep disturbances and may be a component of sleep apnea, in which daytime somnolence and nocturnal wakefulness are common (Chapter 3).

Binge-eating disorder. Binge-eating disorder is a psychiatric illness characterized by uncontrolled episodes of eating, usually in the evening.[21] The patient may respond to treatment with drugs that modulate serotonin.

Infant feeding practices. Infant feeding practices have been related to obesity. Infants fed artificial formula tend to gain more weight per unit time than do breast-fed infants. However, the type of infant feeding (breast or bottle) and rate of weight gain in later childhood do not appear correlated, since weight in the first year has weak predictive value for weight in adolescents unless the child has an overweight parent (see below).

Progressive hyperphagic obesity. A small number of patients begin to be overweight in childhood and then have unrelenting weight gain, usually surpassing 140 kg (300 lb) by 30 years of age. A recent death of a 13-year-old weigh-

Table 5: Genetic Syndromes of Obesity With Hypogonadism and Mental Retardation

Feature	Syndrome	
	Prader-Willi	Bardet-Biedl
Inheritance	Sporadic 2/3 have defect	Autosomal recessive
Stature	Short	Normal, infrequently short
Obesity	Generalized Moderate to severe Onset 1-3 years	Generalized Early onset, 1-2 years
Craniofacial	Narrow bifrontal diameter Almond-shaped eyes Strabismus V-shaped mouth High arched palate	Not distinctive
Limbs	Small hands and feet Hypotonia	Polydactyly
Reproductive status	Primary hypogonadism	Primary hypogonadism
Other features	Enamel hypoplasia Hyperphagia Temper tantrums Nasal speech	
Mental retardation	Mild to moderate	

Alström	Cohen	Carpenter's
Autosomal recessive	Probably autosomal recessive	Autosomal recessive
Normal, infrequently short	Short or tall	Normal
Truncal Early onset, 2-5 years	Truncal Mid childhood, age 5	Truncal Gluteal Mid childhood
Not distinctive	High nasal bridge Arched palate Open mouth Short philtrum	Acrocephaly Flat nasal bridge High arched palate
No abnormalities	Hypotonia Narrow hands and feet	Polydactyly Syndactyly Genu valgum
Hypogonadism in males but not in females	Normal gonadal function or hypogonadotrophic hypogonadism	Secondary hypogonadism
	Dysplastic ears Delayed puberty	
Normal IQ	Mild	Slight

ing 310 kg (680 lb) illustrates the maximal rate of weight gain of nearly 25 kg/year. These patients gain about the same amount of weight year after year. Because approximately 22 kcal/kg is required to maintain an extra kilogram of body weight in an obese individual, the energy requirements in these patients must increase year by year, with the weight gain being driven by excess dietary caloric intake.[2]

Psychologic and Social Factors

Psychologic factors in the development of obesity are widely recognized, although attempts to define a specific personality type that causes obesity have been unsuccessful. One condition linked to weight gain is seasonal affective disorder, which refers to the depression observed during the winter season in people living in the north, where days are short. These patients tend to increase body weight in winter. This can be effectively treated by providing higher-intensity artificial lighting in winter.

Socioeconomic and Ethnic Factors

Obesity is more prevalent in lower socioeconomic groups in the United States and elsewhere (Chapter 1). The inverse relationship of socioeconomic status (SES) and overweight is found in both adults and children. In the Minnesota Heart Study, SES and BMI were inversely related. People of higher SES were more concerned with healthy weight-control practices, including exercise, and tended to eat less fat. In the National Heart, Lung and Blood Institute Growth and Health Study, SES and overweight were strongly associated in white 9- and 10-year-old girls and their mothers, but not in black girls. The association of SES and overweight is much stronger in white women than in black women. Black women of all ages are more obese than white women. Black men are less obese than white men, and socioeconomic factors are much less evident in men. The prevalence of obesity in Hispanic men and women is higher than in whites. The basis for these ethnic differences is unclear. In men, the socioeconomic effects of obesity are weak or absent. This gender difference, and the higher prevalence of overweight in women, suggest important interactions of gender with many factors that influence body fat and fat distribution. The reason for this association is not known.

Genetic and Congenital Disorders

Genetic factors influence obesity in two ways. First, some genes and chromosomal abnormalities are primary factors in the development of obesity. Second, environmental factors act on some genes to cause obesity (Chapter 2). Obesity is also characteristic in several congenital disorders (Table 5).[22] All these syndromes display some degree of reproductive impairment and mental retardation. Prader-Willi syndrome is most common in this group. This abnormality on chromosome 15 q 11.2 is transmitted paternally and produces a 'floppy baby' who usually has trouble feeding. Obesity begins about age 2 and is associated with overeating. Hypogonadism and mental retardation round out the clinical features of this syndrome.

Natural History of Obesity

Individuals can become overweight at any age, but this is more common at certain times. At birth, those who will and those who will not become obese later in life are not distinguished by weight, except for the infants of diabetic mothers, for whom the likelihood of obesity later in life is increased.[1,2] Thus, at birth, a large pool of individuals will eventually become overweight, and a smaller group will never become overweight. I have labeled these pools 'preoverweight' (Figure 2) and 'never overweight', using the NCHS data for prevalence of BMI >25 kg/m^2 as the solid line. Several surveys suggest that one third of overweight adults become overweight before age 20, and two thirds do so after that. Thus, 75% to 80% of adults will become overweight at some time. Between 20% and 25% of the population will display their overweight before age 20, and 50% will do so after age 20.

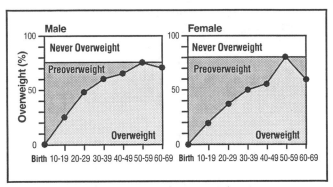

Figure 2: *Natural history of overweight. Because many nonoverweight babies become overweight, this group is labeled preoverweight. About one third of those who become overweight do so before age 20, and two thirds do so after. The remainder are not overweight.*

Some of these overweight individuals will develop clinically significant problems such as diabetes, hypertension, gallbladder disease, or the metabolic syndrome. Thus, the population can be subdivided into four subgroups. The first are the individuals who will never become overweight, although we may only be able to identify them in retrospect. Because most preoverweight people will become overweight, it is important to have as much insight as possible into the risk factors. Table 6 lists many predictors of overweight. These predictors fall into two broad groups: demographic and metabolic. The second are the preoverweight individuals who have a BMI below 25 kg/m². When an individual becomes overweight without clinically significant problems, they manifest 'preclinical overweight'. With the passage of time or a further increase in weight, they may show clinical signs of diabetes, hypertension, gallbladder disease, or dyslipidemia. I call this group 'clinical overweight.' The relationship of one to the other may be depicted as a pyramid (Figure 3).

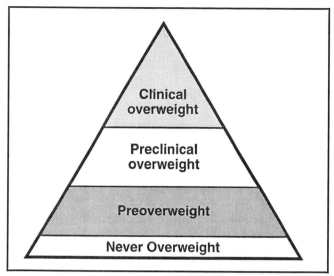

Figure 3: Progression to clinical overweight. Many individuals who become overweight do not have diabetes, hypertension, or other diseases. These are called preclinical overweight. Those who develop clinical disease are clinically overweight.

At the base is the reservoir of never overweight and preoverweight individuals, many of whom will become overweight in their adult life. Some of these will in turn show signs of clinical disease and become clinically overweight. This approach to the natural history of overweight will be used in the approach to treatment outlined in Chapter 5.

Overweight Developing Before Age 10
Prenatal Factors
Caloric intake by the mother may influence body size, shape, and later body composition. Birth weights of identical and fraternal twins have the same correlation (r=.63), indicating that birth weight does not predict future obe-

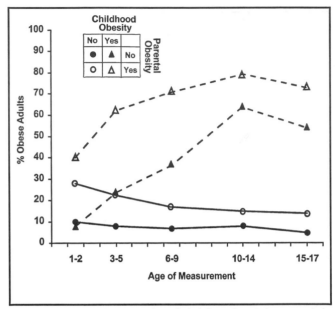

Figure 4: *Effect of parental and childhood weight on weight status during early adulthood. Percentage of overweight adults are plotted in relation to whether the child was overweight at each age and whether the child had one or both overweight parents at the same time. When one parent was overweight, nonoverweight 1- to 2-year-old children had a much greater risk of becoming overweight as an adult, compared to children with no overweight parents. This effect of parental weight status was no longer evident by ages 7 to 9. The effect of parental overweight declined as children entered adolescence, and the tracking of adolescent overweight into early adulthood became much stronger.*[25]

sity. In the first years of life, the correlation of body weight among identical twins begins to converge, rapidly becoming much closer together (r=.9), whereas dizygotic twins diverge during this same period (r=.5). Infants born to diabetic mothers have a higher risk of being overweight as children and adults.[1] Infants who are small-for-dates, short, or have a small head circumference are at higher risk of developing abdominal fatness and other comorbidities associated with obesity later in life.[21]

Infancy Through Age 3

Body weight triples and body fat normally doubles in the first year of life. This increase in body fat in the first year of life is an important predictor of overweight only in infants and young children with overweight parents. An infant above the 85th percentile at age 1 to 3 has a 4-fold increased risk of adult overweight if either parent is overweight, compared with nonoverweight infants. If neither parent is overweight, this infantile overweight does not predict overweight in early adult life (Figure 4). These observations are similar to the older observations suggesting that the risk for adult obesity was 80% for children with two overweight parents, 40% for those with one overweight parent, and less than 10% if neither parent were overweight.[1,2]

Childhood Obesity From Age 3 to 10

An important period of childhood for developing overweight occurs between the ages of 3 and 10 years. *Adiposity rebound* describes the increase in weight of many children as socialization begins around age 5 to 7. About half of the overweight grade school children remained overweight as adults. Moreover, the risk of overweight in adulthood was at least twice as great for overweight children as for nonoverweight children. The risk is 3 to 10 times higher if the child's weight is above the 95th percentile for their age. Parental overweight plays a strong role in this group as well. Nearly 75% of overweight children age 3 to 10 remained overweight in early adulthood if they had one or more overweight parent, compared with 25% to 50% if neither parent were overweight. Overweight 3- to 10-year-olds with an overweight parent thus constitute an ideal group for behavior techniques (chapters 6 and 8). When body weight progressively deviates from

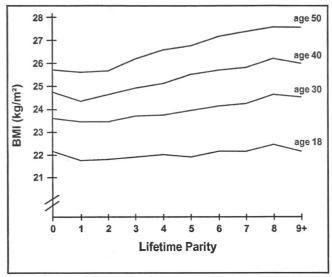

Figure 5: Effect of pregnancy on weight gain. Weight status shifted further with age in women having more children.[29]

the upper limits of normal in this age group, I label it 'progressive obesity'[2]; this is usually severe and lifelong, and is associated with an increase in the number of fat cells.

Overweight Developing in Adolescence and Adult Life

Adolescence

Weight in adolescence becomes a progressively better predictor of adult weight status[25] (Figure 4). In a 55-year follow-up of adolescents, the weight status in adolescence predicted later adverse health events.[27] Adolescents above the 95th percentile had a 5-fold to 20-fold greater likelihood of overweight in adulthood. In contrast with younger ages, parental overweight is less important, or has already had its effect. While 70% to 80% of overweight adolescents with an overweight parent were overweight as young adults, the numbers were only modestly lower (54% to

60%) for overweight adolescents without overweight parents. Despite the importance of childhood and adolescent weight status, however, it remains clear that most overweight individuals develop their problem in adult life.[1,2]

Adult Women

Most overweight women gain their excess weight after puberty. This weight gain may be precipitated by a number of events, including pregnancy, oral contraceptive therapy, and the menopause.

Pregnancy

Weight gain during pregnancy, and the effect of pregnancy on subsequent weight gain, are important events in the weight gain history of women. A few women gain considerable weight during pregnancy, occasionally more than 50 kg. The pregnancy itself may leave a legacy of increased weight, as suggested by one study that evaluated women prospectively between the ages of 18 and 30.[28] Women who remained nulliparous (n=925) were compared with women who had a single pregnancy of 28 weeks' duration during that period and who were at least 12 months postpartum. The primiparas gained 2 to 3 kg more weight and had a greater increase in waist/hip ratio (WHR) compared with the nulliparas during this period. As shown in Figure 5, overweight at each decade increased with increasing parity.[29] The overall risk of weight gain associated with child-bearing after age 25, however, is quite modest for American women.[30]

Oral Contraceptives

Oral contraceptive use may initiate weight gain in some women, although this effect is diminished with the low-dose estrogen pills. One study evaluated 49 healthy women initiating treatment with low-dose oral contraceptives (30 mg ethinyl estradiol plus 75 mg gestodene). Anthropometric measurements before and after the initiation of this formulation were used to compare 31 age- and weight-matched women.[31] Baseline BMI, percent fat, percent water, and WHR did not change significantly after six cycles in the birth control pill users. A similar number of women gained weight in both groups (30.6% of users, 35.4% of controls). The typical weight gain in the pill user group was only 0.5 kg, but the small weight gain in these women was attributable to the accumulation of fat, not body water. Approximately 20% of women in both groups lost weight.

Menopause

Weight gain and changes in fat distribution occur after the menopause. The decline in estrogen and progesterone secretion alters fat cell biology so that central fat deposition increases (Chapter 1). Central or abdominal fat deposition (as estimated clinically from waist circumference or WHR) is an important determinant of cardiovascular risk.

Estrogen replacement therapy does not prevent the weight gain, although it may minimize fat redistribution.[32] A prospective study of 63 early postmenopausal women compared 34 who initiated continuous estrogen and progesterone therapy to the remaining women who refused it. Body weight and fat mass increased significantly in both the treatment (73.2 to 75.6 kg) and the control groups (71.5 to 73.5 kg). However, WHR increased significantly only in the control group (0.80 to 0.85). Caloric and macronutrient intake did not change in either group. A 2-year trial with estrogen in postmenopausal women also showed an increase in body fat.[33]

Adult Men

The transition from an active lifestyle during the teens and early 20s to a more sedentary lifestyle thereafter is associated with weight gain in many men. A rise in body weight continues through the adult years until the sixth decade (Figure 2). After ages 55 to 64, relative weight remains stable and then begins to decline. Evidence from the Framingham Study and studies of men in the armed services suggests that men have become progressively heavier for height during this century (Chapter 2).

Weight Stability and Weight Cycling

Body weight varies throughout the day as food is eaten and then metabolized. Body weight also varies from day to day, week to week, and over longer intervals. Understanding these fluctuations and their relationship to more significant weight cycling related to dieting and regain (yo-yo dieting) is important in understanding obesity.[35] Williamson examined changes in weight over time.[34] Adults under age 55 tend to gain weight, and those over 55 tend to lose it. The youngest adults gain the most weight, and the oldest adults lose the most. Women have significantly greater variation in their weight over 10 years than do men. A 25% weight gain was found in 2.9% of men aged 25 to 44, compared with 6.5% of women in the same age group. In the middle-age range, the numbers with weight gain of 25% had dropped by nearly half: 1.8% of men age 45 to 64, compared with 2.9% of women in the same age group. Weight loss of 25% or more in Americans age 65 to 74 was higher in women (6.5%) than in men (2.2%). The likelihood of a significant weight gain was substantially higher in the overweight than in those of normal weight in the younger age groups.[34] Because the incidence of significant weight gain is more common in young adults, these are a prime target for preventive measures.

Weight cycling associated with dieting is popularly known as yo-yo dieting.[35] Weight cycling refers to the downs and ups in weight that often happen to people who diet, lose weight, stop dieting, and regain the weight they lost and sometimes more. The possibility that loss and regain is more detrimental than staying heavy has been hotly debated. In a review of the literature between 1964 and 1994, a group of experts concluded that most studies did not support any adverse effects on metabolism associated with weight cycling. Also, little or no data supported the contention that it is more difficult to lose weight a second time after regaining weight from a previous therapeutic approach. Most researchers agree that weight cycling neither necessarily increases body fat, nor adversely affects blood pressure, glucose metabolism, or lipid concentrations.

References

1.   Bray GA: The syndromes of obesity: an endocrine approach. In: DeGroot LJ, Besser M, Burger HB, et al, eds. *Endocrinology*. Philadelphia, WB Saunders, 1995, pp 2624-2662.

2.   Bray GA: *The Obese Patient: Major Problems in Internal Medicine*, 9th ed. Philadelphia, WB Saunders, 1976.

3.   Bray GA, Fisler JS, York DA: Neuroendocrine control of the development of obesity: understanding gained from studies of experimental animal models. *Front Neuroendocrinol* 1990;11:128-181.

4.   Bray GA, Gallagher TF Jr: Manifestations of hypothalamic obesity in man: a comprehensive investigation of eight patients and a review of the literature. *Medicine (Baltimore)* 1975;54:301-330.

5.   Wajchenberg BL, Bosco A, Marone MM, et al: Estimation of body fat and lean tissue distribution by dual energy X-ray absorptiometry and abdominal body fat evaluation by computed tomography in Cushing's disease. *J Clin Endocrinol Metab* 1995;80:2791-2794.

6.   Zelissen PM, Koppenschaar HP: The dexamethasone-corticotropin releasing hormone (CRH) test differentiates accurately between Cushing's syndrome and central morbid obesity. *Obes Res* 1997;5:88S.

7.   Kiddy DS, Sharp PS, White DM, et al: Differences in clinical and endocrine features between obese and non-obese subjects with polycystic ovary syndrome: an analysis of 263 consecutive cases. *Clin Endocrinol (Oxf)* 1990;32:213-220.

8.   Lonn L, Johansson G, Sjostrom L, et al: Body composition and tissue distributions in growth hormone deficient adults before and after growth hormone treatment. *Obes Res* 1996;4:45-54.

9.   Loprinzi CL, Schaid DJ, Dose AM, et al: Body-composition changes in patients who gain weight while receiving megestrol acetate. *J Clin Oncol* 1993;11:152-154.

10.   United Kingdom Prospective Diabetes Study Group: United Kingdom Prospective Diabetes Study 24: a 6-year, randomized, controlled trial comparing sulfonylurea, insulin, and metformin therapy in patients with newly diagnosed type 2 diabetes that could not be controlled with diet therapy. *Ann Intern Med* 1998;128:165-175.

11. The Diabetes Control and Complications Trial Research Group: Weight gain associated with intensive therapy in the diabetes control and complications trial. *Diabetes Care* 1988;11:567-573.

12. Flegal KM, Troiano RP, Pamuk ER, et al: The influence of smoking cessation on the prevalence of overweight in the United States. *N Engl J Med* 1995;333:1165-1170.

13. Prentice AM, Jebb SA: Obesity in Britain: gluttony or sloth? *BMJ* 1995;311:437-439.

14. Kromhout D: Changes in energy and macronutrients in 871 middle-aged men during 10 years of follow-up (the Zutphen study). *Am J Clin Nutr* 1983;37:287-294.

15. U.S. Department of Health and Human Services: *Physical Activity and Health: A Report of the Surgeon General.* Atlanta, Centers for Disease Control and Prevention, National Center for Chronic Disease Prevention and Health Promotion, 1996.

16. Bouchard CA, Tremblay A, Despres JP, et al: The response to long-term overfeeding in identical twins. *N Engl J Med* 1990;322:1477-1482.

17. Lawson OJ, Williamson DA, Champagne CM, et al: The association of body weight, dietary intake, and energy expenditure with dietary restraint and disinhibition. *Obes Res* 1995;3:153-161.

18. Williamson DA, Lawson OJ, Brooks ER, et al: Association of body mass with dietary restraint and disinhibition. *Appetite* 1995;25:31-41.

19. Jenkins DJ, Wolever TM, Vuksan V, et al: Nibbling versus gorging: metabolic advantages of increased meal frequency. *N Engl J Med* 1989;321:929-934.

20. Bray GA, Popkin BM: Dietary fat intake does affect obesity! *Am J Clin Nutr* 1998, in press.

21. Yanovski SZ, Gormally JF, Leser MS, et al: Binge eating disorder affects outcome of comprehensive very-low-calorie diet treatment. *Obes Res* 1994;2:205-212.

22. Bray GA: Obesity. In: King RA, Rotter JI, Motulsky AG, eds. *The Genetic Basis of Common Diseases.* New York, Oxford University Press, 1992, pp 507-528.

23. Chagnon YC, Perusse L, Bouchard C: The human obesity gene map: the 1997 update. *Obes Res* 1998;6:76-92.

24. Barker DJ, Hales CN, Fall CH, et al: Type 2 (non-insulin-dependent) diabetes mellitus, hypertension and hyperlipidaemia (syndrome X): relation to reduced fetal growth. *Diabetologia* 1993;36:62-67.

25. Whitaker RC, Wright JA, Pepe MS, et al: Predicting obesity in young adulthood from childhood and parental obesity. *N Engl J Med* 1997;337:869-873.

26. Braddon FE, Rodgers B, Wadsworth ME, et al: Onset of obesity in a 36 year birth cohort study. *Br Med J (Clin Res Ed)* 1986;293:299-303.

27. Must A, Jacques PF, Dallal GE, et al: Long-term morbidity and mortality of overweight adolescents. A follow-up of the Harvard Growth Study of 1922 to 1935. *N Engl J Med* 1992;327:1350-1355.

28. Smith DE, Lewis CE, Caveny JL, et al: Longitudinal changes in adiposity associated with pregnancy. The CARDIA Study. Coronary Artery Risk Development in Young Adults Study. *JAMA* 1994;271:1747-1751.

29. Brown JE, Kaye SA, Folsom AR: Parity-related weight change in women. *Int J Obes Relat Metab Disord* 1992;16:627-631.

30. Williamson DF, Madans J, Pamuk E, et al: A prospective study of childbearing and 10-year weight gain in US white women 25 to 45 years of age. *Int J Obes Relat Metab Disord* 1994;18:561-569.

31. Reubinoff BE, Grubstein A, Meirow D, et al: Effects of low-dose estrogen oral contraceptives on weight, body composition, and fat distribution in young women. *Fertil Steril* 1995;63:516-521.

32. Aloia JF, Vaswani A, Russo L, et al: The influence of menopause and hormonal replacement therapy on body cell mass and body fat mass. *Am J Obstet Gynecol* 1995;172:896-900.

33. Haarbo J, Christiansen C: Treatment-induced cyclic variations in serum lipids, lipoproteins, and apolipoproteins after 2 years of combined hormone replacement therapy: exaggerated cyclic variations in smokers. *Obstet Gynecol* 1992;80:639-644.

34. Williamson DF: Descriptive epidemiology of body weight and weight change in U.S. adults. *Ann Intern Med* 1993;119:646-649.

35. National Task Force on the Prevention and Treatment of Obesity: Weight cycling. *JAMA* 1994;272:1196-1202.

Chapter 5

Clinical Evaluation and Introduction to Treatment of Overweight

"The human body is composed
Of head and limbs and torso
Kept slim by gents
At great expense
By ladies even more so."

— Ogden Nash

The previous four chapters examined overweight from a diagnostic and pathophysiologic perspective. This chapter and the remaining chapters focus on treatment. This chapter briefly summarizes the points made so far, and provides an overview of remaining chapters.

The Realities of Overweight

Overweight is a chronic, stigmatized disease that is increasing in prevalence. The 33% of the American population who are now overweight represent 58 million people, a 30% increase in the last 15 years. The social disapproval of obesity and the lengths people go to prevent or reverse it fuels a $50 billion a year set of industries. Nearly 65% of American women consider themselves overweight, and even more (66% to 75%) want to weigh less. The figures for men are somewhat less. More than 50% of the women with a body mass index (BMI) below 21 kg/m² (normal

131

weight) want to weigh less. This individual perception of a 'desirable' weight for them indicates the degree of both the stigmatization for those who are not 'thin' and the drive to lose weight.

The cultural expectations for thinness are evident in the decreasing weight of the Miss America contestants since 1950, and in the centerfolds of Playboy magazine. The stigma of obesity is also evident in the general public disapproval of corpulence, and in the disapproving moral attitudes of many health-care professionals. For example, mental health workers are more likely to assign negative psychologic symptoms to the obese than to normal-weight people. Nursing, medical, and ancillary health-care personnel also carry these negative stereotypes. Sensitivity training for health professionals dealing with overweight patients is important in any office or clinic offering treatment for obesity.

As noted in Chapter 4, overweight has many causes. The natural history of obesity indicates that it occurs gradually. Although overweight in childhood carries a serious adverse prognosis, particularly if parents are overweight, nearly two thirds of overweight adults developed their problem in adult life. The risk for obesity with advancing age is illustrated in Chapter 4, Figure 2, which shows the proportion of American men and women with BMI >25 at various decades of life. Because the proportion increases until the sixth decade, those whose BMI is <25 are considered preoverweight; those with BMI >25 and <30 are considered preclinically overweight; and those with BMI >30 are considered clinically overweight.

Results from most long-term clinical studies of treatment for overweight patients show a high prevalence of weight regain. In the Institute of Medicine report *Weighing the Options*, for those who achieved weight loss, more than one third of the weight typically was regained within 1 year, and nearly all within 5 years.[1] Despite this gloomy

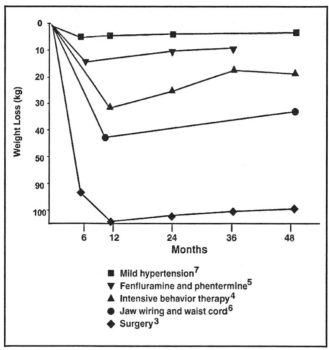

Figure 1: Comparison of 3- to 4-year weight losses. Each line represents a single study showing that weight loss varies greatly among treatments, and that maximum weight loss usually occurs in the first year. Long-term weight reduction is possible when the treatment is continuous, as in all of these studies.

report, many long-term successes have occurred.[2-7] A study of successful weight maintainers showed no differences from unsuccessful weight maintainers in reported level of energy expenditure from exercise. However, those who successfully maintained weight loss showed greater control of fat intake, which included avoiding fried foods and substituting low-fat foods for high-fat foods. Several other programs have also reported long-term weight

133

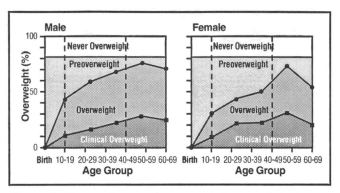

Figure 2: Comparison of preoverweight, preclinical over-weight, and clinical overweight as a percentage of respective age groups.

loss maintenance, especially in children.[2] Figure 1 compares five studies that reported data for 4 years. The largest weight loss with the greatest maintenance was in individuals who underwent surgery[3] (Chapter 10). Behavior therapy produced modest weight loss unless actively continued[4] (Chapter 6). Pharmacologic therapy produced an 11% weight loss over 3.5 years[5] (Chapter 9). Most intriguingly, the second-best weight loss was produced by a nylon waist cord after initial weight loss was produced by jaw wiring[6] (Chapter 10). Diet alone in a treatment program for high blood pressure produced only a small effect.[7]

Overweight, central or visceral fat, weight gain after age 20, and a sedentary lifestyle all increase health risks and increase economic costs of obesity. Intentional weight loss by overweight individuals, on the other hand, reduces these risks (Chapter 3). Although data are not yet available, researchers widely believe that long-term intentional weight loss lowers overall mortality, particularly from diabetes, gallbladder disease, hypertension, heart disease, and some types of cancer.

Data from the National Center for Health Statistics[16] are plotted in Figure 2 to show the prevalence of overweight (BMI >25 kg/m^2) and obesity (BMI >30 kg/m^2) to show the transition phases. The percentage of the population who are preoverweight falls as people move into the preclinical and clinical overweight categories.

Clinical Evaluation of Overweight Patients

This section addresses clinical evaluation of overweight patients,[8,9] and then reviews criteria for successful outcomes of treatment and goals of preventing progression from preoverweight to preclinical and clinical overweight.

Both clinical and laboratory information are needed to evaluate overweight patients. The criteria correspond with those of the U.S. Preventive Services Task Force,[10] but rely more heavily on the American Obesity Association[11] and World Health Organization reports.[12] This approach focuses on characterizing the type of obesity and emphasizing prevention of progression. This approach assumes many types of overweight individuals, with different degrees of associated risk. Some types of overweight can be distinguished, and the relative risks identified. The importance of evaluating all types of overweight has increased as the epidemic of obesity has worsened and the number of potential treatments has increased.

Several reports provide guidance for this evaluation. These reports come from the American Obesity Association,[11] the American Association of Clinical Endocrinologists,[13] and the World Health Organization Consultation.[12]

Body Weight

Table 1 provides a form to record relevant clinical and laboratory data when evaluating an overweight patient. This helps categorize the patient as preoverweight, preclinically overweight, or clinically overweight. Accurate measurement of height and weight is the initial step in the clinical assessment of overweight.[14,15] The

Table 1: Clinical and Laboratory Data for Evaluating Overweight Patients

Name:

Age:

Date of Birth:

Measured Data

Height (in or cm):	____ in	____ cm
Weight (lb or kg)	____ lb	____ kg
Weight at age 20	____ lb	____ kg
Waist circumference	____ in	____ cm
Hip circumference	____ in	____ cm
Blood pressure (mm Hg)	systolic	diastolic
Triglycerides	____ mg/dL	____ mmol
HDL cholesterol	____ mg/dL	____ mmol
Fasting glucose	____ mg/dL	____ mmol
Sleep apnea	yes	no
Medications that increase weight	yes	no
Chief cause (if known)	____	

most practical way to evaluate the degree of overweight is BMI. This index is calculated as the body weight (kg) divided by the stature (height [m]) squared (wt/ht^2), and can be obtained from Figure 3, or from Chapter 1, Table 5. BMI correlates well with body fat, and is relatively unaffected by height.

BMI shows a curvilinear relationship to risk (Figure 4). Several levels of risk can be identified. These cutpoints are derived from data collected on Caucasians.

Identifying Number:

Date:

Date of Birth:

Derived Data

BMI (kg/m^2): ___

Weight gain since age 20 ___

Waist circumference/hip circumference (WHR) ___

Whether they accurately apply to other ethnic groups is not yet clear, but until other criteria become available, they are the best we have. Data from Hispanics and African Americans suggest that increased body fat carries a greater risk of diabetes, but has less impact on heart disease (Chapter 3). Figure 4 also identifies cutpoints to separate preoverweight from preclinical overweight and clinical overweight, using BMI alone (Chapter 4). After treatment begins, regular measurement of body weight

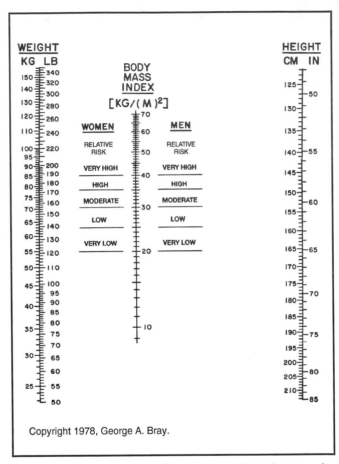

Figure 3: Nomogram for determining BMI. Place a ruler or other straight edge between the body weight in kilograms or pounds (without clothes) located on the left-hand line and the height in centimeters or in inches (without shoes) located on the right-hand line. BMI is read from the middle of the scale in metric units. (Copyright 1978, George A. Bray, MD. Used with permission.)

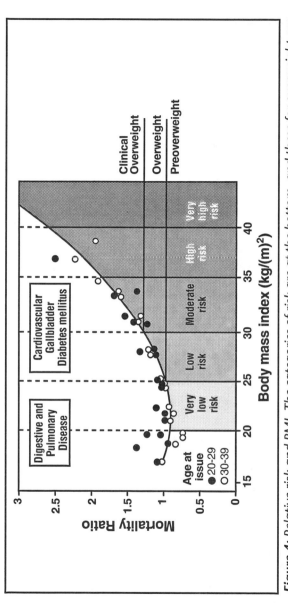

Figure 4: *Relative risk and BMI. The categories of risk are at the bottom, and these for overweight are on the right. Individuals with a BMI below 25 are preoverweight, those with a BMI 25 to 30 are preclinical overweight, and those above 30 are clinically overweight. Copyright 1997, George A. Bray.*

139

Table 2: Risk Associated With Different Levels of Central Fat

BMI Adjustment if Initial BMI is Between 22 and 29

Men	Waist circumference	in
		cm
	WHR	
Women	Waist circumference	in
		cm
	WHR	

BMI is evaluated and adjusted for the added risk
of central fat for indiviuals with BMI below 30 kg/m².

Table 3: Risk Associated With Weight Gain

	Weight Gain Since Age 20 in kg		
	<5	5-10	>10
Risk	Low	Moderate	High
Risk score	0	+1	+2

is one important way to follow the progress of any treatment program.

Regional Fat Distribution

Visceral fat and central fatness can be evaluated by several methods (Chapter 1). The most accurate are computed tomography (CT) or magnetic resonance imaging (MRI), but these are expensive and not generally available for

	Risk	
Low	**Moderate**	**High**
	Risk Score	
0	+2	+4
<37	37-40	>40
<94	94-102	>102
<.90	.90-1.00	>1.00
<32	32-35	>35
<80	80-88	>88
<.75	.75-.85	>.85

this purpose. Waist circumference or the ratio of waist circumference to hip circumference (WHR) are the most practical clinical alternatives. Waist circumference is measured with a flexible tape placed horizontally at the level of the natural waist line or narrowest part of the torso as seen anteriorly.[15] Hip circumference is measured horizontally at the maximum circumference, including the maximum extension of the buttocks posteriorly. A nomogram for calculating WHR is shown in Figure 5. Figure 6 displays the risk associated with WHR across various ages.

Table 2 shows the risk associated with different waist circumferences or WHR. Measuring changing waist circumference is another good tool for following the progress of weight loss. It is particularly valuable when patients become more physically active. Physical activity may slow loss of muscle mass and thus slow weight loss while fat continues to be mobilized. Waist circumference can help in making this distinction. Table 3 presents waist circum-

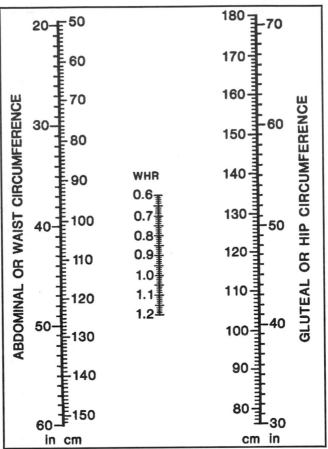

Figure 5: *Nomogram for determining WHR. Place a straight edge between the column for waist circumference and the column for hip circumference. Read the ratio from the point where this straight edge crosses the WHR line. The waist circumference is the smallest circumference below the rib cage and above the umbilicus, and the hip circumference is the largest circumference at posterior extension of the buttocks. (Copyright 1987, George A. Bray, MD. Reproduced with permission).*

142

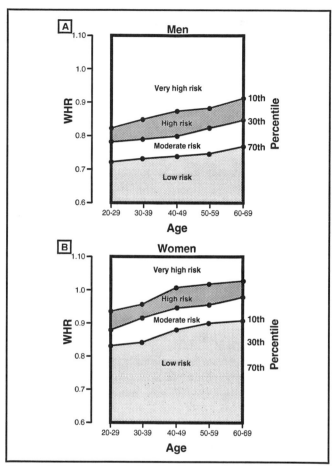

Figure 6: Percentiles for fat distribution in men and women. The percentiles for the ratio of abdominal circumference to hip circumference are depicted for men (A) and women (B) by age group. Relative risk for these percentiles is indicated based on available information. (Plotted from tabular data in the Canadian Standardized Test of Fitness, Third Edition, 1986. Copyright 1987, George A. Bray, MD. Used with permission.)

ferences for men and women equivalent to WHR values for low, moderate, and high risk. As with BMI, the relationship of central fat to risk factors for health varies among populations as well as within them. Japanese Americans and Indians from South Asia have relatively more visceral fat and are thus at higher risk for a given BMI or total body fat than are Caucasians living in the same region. Thus, the risk assigned to waist circumference or WHR in Table 2 must be tempered by the group to which it is applied. Even though the BMI may be below 25 kg/m^2, central fat may be increased and, thus, adjustment of BMI for central adiposity is important, particularly with BMI between 22 and 29 kg/m^2.

Weight Gain

Weight gain is associated with increased risk to health (Table 3). Three categories of weight gain are identified: <5 kg (<11 lb); 5 to 10 kg (11 to 22 lb); and >10 kg (>22 lb). The adjusted score can be used to calculate risk-adjusted body mass index.

Sedentary Lifestyle

A sedentary lifestyle also increases the risk of early death. Individuals with no regular physical activity are at higher risk than individuals with modest levels of physical activity. This is addressed more fully in Chapter 8.

Etiologic Factors

Etiologic factors and the natural history of obesity should be identified, if possible.[9,17] These are described in detail in Chapter 4, and should be noted on the form for laboratory data (Table 1) if they are identified. The algorithm in Figure 7 helps identify etiologic factors.[17] Questions begin in the upper left-hand corner. A positive answer at any point leads to suggestions for clinical evaluation. For example, once overweight has been established, the possibility of hypertension is addressed.

If hypertension is present, the clinician should search for clinical signs of Cushing's syndrome. If these are present, a urinary free cortisol test is recommended, followed by dexamethasone-CRH test if indicated (Chapter 4). If Cushing's syndrome is not suspected, a hypertension work-up is suggested. In turn, the algorithm directs a search for clinical clues of hypothyroidism, glucose intolerance, dyslipidemia, hypoventilation sleep-apnea syndrome, CNS lesions, polycystic ovary syndrome, and congestive heart failure.

Acanthosis nigricans deserves a brief comment. This is a clinical condition with increased pigmentation in the folds of the neck, along the exterior surface of the distal extremities, and over the knuckles. It may signify increased insulin resistance or malignancy, and should be evaluated. At each point, the algorithm suggests further work-up when appropriate.

Introduction to Treatment
Risk-Benefit Assessment

Once the work-up for etiologic and complicating factors is complete, the risk associated with elevated BMI can be evaluated. Several algorithms can be used for this purpose.[11-13,18]

I will use the method shown in Figure 8.[18] BMI is determined (Table 1). Initial BMI provides the first level of risk. Individuals with a BMI below 25 kg/m² are at very low risk but, nonetheless, nearly half of those in this category at ages 20 to 25 will become overweight by age 60 to 69 (Chapter 4). Thus, a large group of preoverweight individuals need preventive strategies. Risk rises with a BMI above 25 kg/m². The presence of complicating factors further increases this risk. Thus, an attempt at a quantitative estimate of these complicating factors is important.

The proposed method for adjusting the BMI for other risk factors is shown in Table 4, which provides the adjustment scores for central fat distribution using waist cir-

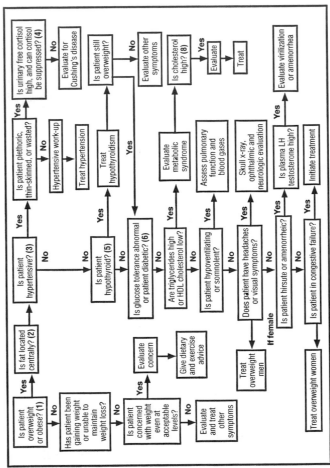

Figure 7:
Algorithm for evaluating overweight patients.

(1) Overweight is defined as BMI between 25 and 30 kg/m²; obesity is BMI above 30 kg/m².

(2) Fat distribution is defined by waist circumference or the ratio of waist circumference divided by hip circumference (Table 4).

(3) Blood pressure readings were taken with a large cuff that encircles 75% of the arm.

(4) Dexamethasone suppression test: suppression is a cortisol less than 3 µg/dL (80 nmol/L) at 8:00 a.m., 9 hours after 1 mg of dexamethasone orally. If not suppressed, evaluate for Cushing's disease.

(5) Thyroid Function:

	Serum Thyroxine (corrected)		Serum Thyrotropin
	(µg/dL)	*(nmol/L)*	*(µU/mL=mU/L)*
Possible hyperthyroidism	12	154	<2
Normal	5.5-12.0	71-154	2-7
Borderline hypothyroidism	4.0-5.5	51-71	7-10
Hypothyroidism	4.0	51	>10

In the presence of severe illness, a low serum thyroxine must be interpreted cautiously; it may be a bad prognostic sign, but does not indicate hypothyroidism unless TSH is elevated.

(6) The diagnosis of diabetes in nonpregnant adults is based on the following:

• *Unequivocal hyperglycemia and classic symptoms of diabetes mellitus*

• *Fasting venous plasma glucose >126 mg/dL (7.0 mmol/L)*

• *Fasting plasma glucose >126 mg/dL (7.0 mmol/L) at some point between 0 and 2 hours, and 2 hours after an oral glucose tolerance test with 75 g glucose (or, for children, 1.75 g/kg of ideal body weight, not to exceed 75 g)*

(7) Triglycerides >2.3 mmol

Triglycerides	**mg/dL**
Normal	<200
Borderline high	200-400
High	400-1000
Very high	>1000

(8) LDL cholesterol: for total cholesterol >200 mg/dL, determine LDL cholesterol and evaluate risk.

	Diet Therapy	Consider Drugs	Goal of Treatment
Without CHD and <2 risk factors	>160	>190	<160
Without CHD and 2 or more risk factors	>130	>160	<130
With CHD	>100	>130	<100

Risk factors include: family history of premature coronary heart disease (age <55); hypertension; cigarette smoking; diabetes mellitus; and low HDL cholesterol (<0.9 mmol/L or <35 mg/dL). An HDL cholesterol >60 mg/dL (1.6 mmol/L) is protective.

cumference interpreted in light of the considerations about ethnic variability. Waist circumference identifies the adjustment score, which should be noted on the appropriate line of Table 4. Table 4 also provides space for the adjustment scores for each of several other obesity-related metabolic and clinical variables already recorded in Table 1. The scores for each are recorded on the right-hand side and added to the patient's BMI (top line) to obtain the adjusted score.

Treatments for obesity can be risky, as evidenced by the results from the past 100 years (Table 5). Treatment must be applied over the long term, hence the emphasis on risk-benefit and safety. Each significant treatment has been associated with a therapeutic disaster. This must temper enthusiasm for new treatments unless the risk is very

Table 4: Risk-Adjusted BMI for Metabolic Variables

Score	| Adjustment Scores			Adjustment Score
	0	+2	+4	
BMI				____
Weight gain since age 18 (kg)	<5	5-15	>15	____
Triglyceride/ HDL cholesterol (mg/dL)	<5	5-8	>8	____
Blood pressure (mm Hg)	<140/ <90	140-160/ 90-100	>160/ >100	____
Fasting glucose (mg/dL)	<95	96-126	>126	____
Waist circumference, inches (cm)	(f) <32 (81) (m) <37 (94)	32-35 (81-89) 37-40 (94-102)	>35 (89) >40 (102)	____
Sleep apnea	Absent		Present	____
Physical activity	Regular activity	Sedentary		____
Risk-Adjusted Index				____

low. Because obesity is stigmatized, any treatment approved by the FDA will be used for cosmetic purposes by preoverweight people who suffer the stigma of obesity. Thus, drugs to treat obesity must have very high safety profiles.

When the adjusted score is determined, overall risk assessment and treatment goals can be evaluated (Table 6).

Table 5: Disasters With Drug Treatments for Obesity

Date	Drug	Outcome
1893	Thyroid	Hyperthyroidism
1933	Dinitrophenol	Cataracts, neuropathy
1937	Amphetamine	Addiction
1967	Rainbow pills (digitalis, diuretics)	Death
1971	Aminorex	Pulmonary hypertension
1997	Fenfluramine/ phentermine	Valvular insufficiency

Risk-adjusted BMI is divided into 5-unit intervals, just as in Figure 4. Risk, goals, and potential treatment strategies are noted opposite each of these intervals. Low levels of comorbid risks reduce the impact of any BMI, whereas high levels of comorbid risk augment the effect of BMI. Using the adjusted score, selection or rank ordering of treatments is possible, as shown in Figure 8.

Patient Readiness

Before initiating any treatment, establishing the patient's readiness to make changes is important. A series of questions developed by Brownell[19] can assess this. These are provided in Appendix A, The Dieting Readiness Test.

When counseling patients who are ready to lose weight, accommodation of their individual needs as well as ethnic factors, age, and other differences is essential. The approach outlined above is not rigid and must be used to help guide clinical decision making, and not serve as an alternative to considering individual factors in developing a treatment plan. Because of increasing complications

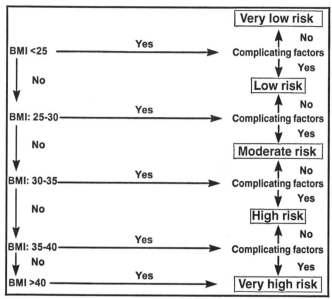

Figure 8: Risk classification algorithm. The patient is categorized based on initial BMI. The presence of complicating factors shift risk up or down. (Copyright 1987, George A. Bray, MD. Used with permission.)[18]

of obesity, more aggressive efforts at therapy should be directed at people in each of the successively higher risk classifications.

Patient-Doctor Expectations

The realities of treatment for obesity often conflict with patients' expectations. Patients were asked to give the weights they wanted to achieve in several categories, from their dream weight to a weight loss that would leave them disappointed. These are listed in column 2 of Table 7.[20] Patients then participated in a weight loss program. The percentage achieving each goal is listed in the right-hand column. None of the patients achieved

Table 6: Strategy for Using Body Mass Index to Select Treatment for Overweight Patients

Body Mass Index	# of Risk Factors	High Waist Circumference	Risk Category	Treat Risk Factors
<25	0	No	Very low	No
	0	Yes	Low	No
	≥1	Y or N	Moderate	Yes
25-<29.9	0	No	Low	No
	0	Yes	Moderate	No
	≥1	Y or N	Moderate	Yes
30-<34.9	0	Y or N	Moderate	No
	≥1	Y or N	High	Yes
<35	0	Y or N	High	No
	≥1	Y or N	Very high	Yes

Risk factors:
Diabetes; impaired glucose tolerance or fasting glucose 110-126 mg/dL
HDL cholesterol: M <35 mg/dL TG >200
F <45 mg/dL TG >200
Treated hypertension or blood pressure >140/>90

High waist circumference:
M >102 cm (40 in)
F >88 cm (35 in)

their dream weight, which was an average 38% below baseline. Nearly half failed to achieve even a weight loss outcome that would disappoint them. Desirability from a cosmetic standpoint almost always conflicts with realistically achievable goals. This mismatch between patient expectations and the realities of weight loss pro-

Consider as Treatment for Overweight

Diet	Exercise	Behavior Therapy	Pharmaco-therapy	Sur-gery
Advice for healthy living			-	-
+	+	+	-	-
+	+	+	-	-
+	+	+	-	-
+	+	+	±	-
+	+	+	+	-
+	+	+	+	-
+	+	+	+	-
+	+	+	+	±
+	+	+	+	+

vides clinicians and their patients with an important challenge as they begin treatment. A weight loss goal of 5% to 15% can be achieved by most patients and is reasonable.

One complaint about treatments for obesity is that they frequently fail, and thus are 'no good.' An alternative

Table 7: Weight Goals of 60 Overweight Women[20]

Imagined Goal	Weight loss (kg) to achieve goal (%)	% of subjects achieving goal
Dream weight	37.7 (38)	0
Happy weight	31.1 (31)	9%
Acceptable weight	24.9 (25)	24%
Disappointed weight	17.2 (17)	20%
Below disappointed weight	—	47%
Baseline weight = 99.1 kg		

interpretation may be better. Overweight is not curable, but can be treated in many ways. When treatment is stopped, weight is regained. This is similar to what happens in patients with hypertension who stop taking their antihypertensive drugs, and in patients with high cholesterol who stop taking their hypocholesterolemic drugs. In each case, blood pressure or cholesterol rises. Like overweight, these chronic diseases have not been cured, but rather palliated. When treatment is stopped, the risk factor recurs. A weight decrease of 5% to 15% from baseline improves most comorbidities associated with overweight.[1] Patients who are ready to lose weight and have a reasonable expectation of weight loss are ready to begin. An ideal outcome is a return of body weight to normal range, with no weight gain thereafter. This is rarely achieved and is unrealistic for patients; thus, they need guidance in accepting a realistic goal, usually a loss of 5% to 15%.[1] A satisfactory outcome is a maintenance of body weight over the ensuing years. A good outcome would be a loss of 5% to 15% of initial body weight and regain no faster than the increase in body weight of the population. Patients who achieve this should be applauded. An excellent outcome would be weight loss of more than 15% of body weight. An unsatisfactory outcome is a loss of less than 5% with regain above the population weight.

Treatment Strategies by Age Group

After evaluating a patient and deciding that he or she is ready to lose weight, the patient can be placed in one of the categories based on the risk-adjusted body mass index. The basic approaches to prevention and treatment are based on this characterization and the patient's age.

Age 1-10

Table 8 shows the strategies available for overweight and obese children. A variety of genetic factors can enhance obesity in this age group, which also contains a high percentage of preoverweight individuals. Identifying individuals at highest risk for becoming overweight in adult life allows for a focus on preventive strategies. Among these strategies are the need to develop patterns of physical activity and good eating habits, including a lower fat intake and a lower energy-density diet. Table 9 lists some predictors for developing overweight. Some of these are evident in children; others are not until adult life. For growing children, medications should be used to directly treat the comorbidities. Drugs for weight loss are generally inappropriate until the patient reaches adult height, and surgical intervention should only be considered after consultation with medical and surgical experts.

Age 11-50

Table 10 outlines the available strategies for overweight and obese adults. Since nearly two thirds of preoverweight individuals move into the overweight and

Table 8: Therapeutic Strategies, Age 1-10

Age	Predictors of Overweight	Preoverweight at Risk
1-10	Positive family history	Family counseling
	Genetic defects (dysmorphic-PWS; Bardet-Biedl; Cohen)	Reduce inactivity
	Hypothalamic injury	
	Low metabolic rate	
	Diabetic mother	

obese categories in this age range, this range is quantitatively most important. Preventive strategies should be used for patients with predictors of weight gain (Table 9). These should include advice on lifestyle changes, including increased physical activity, which would benefit al-

Table 9: Predictors of Weight Gain

- Parental overweight
- Lower socioeconomic status
- Smoking cessation
- Low level of physical activity
- Low metabolic rate
- Childhood overweight
- Heavy babies
- Lack of maternal knowledge of child's sweet-eating habits
- Recent marriage
- Multiple births

Therapeutic Strategies

Preclinical Overweight	Clinical Overweight
Family behavior therapy	Treat comorbidities
Exercise	Exercise
Low-fat/low-energy-dense diet	Low-fat/low-energy-dense diet

most all adults, and good dietary practices, including a diet lower in saturated fat.

For patients in the overweight category, behavior strategies should be added to these lifestyle strategies. This is particularly important for overweight adolescents, because good 10-year data show that intervention for this group can reduce the degree of overweight in adult life.[2] Data on the efficacy of behavior programs carried out in controlled settings show that weight losses average nearly 10% in trials lasting more than 16 weeks. The limitation is the likelihood of regaining weight once the behavior treatment ends, although as shown in Figure 1,[4] the long-term behavior therapy study did provide long-term weight loss.

Medication should be seriously considered for clinically overweight individuals in this group (see Chapter 8). Two strategies can be used. The first is to use drugs to treat each comorbidity, ie, individually treating diabetes, hypertension, dyslipidemia, and sleep apnea with appropriate medications. Alternatively, or in addition, patients with an adjusted BMI above 30 kg/m^2 could be treated with antiobesity drugs. All available drugs are

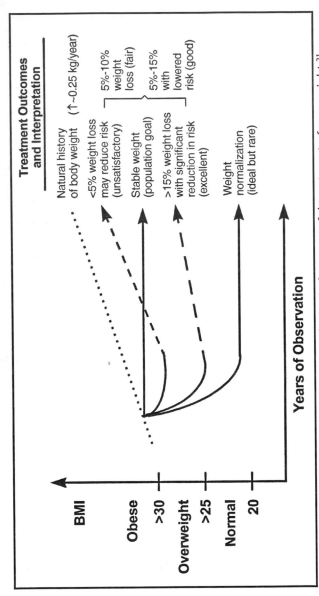

Figure 9: Natural history of weight gain and criteria for successful treatment of overweight.[21]

158

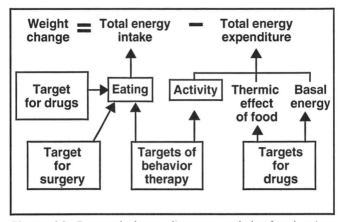

Figure 10: *Energy balance diagram and the focal points where treatments for overweight can be targeted.*

appetite suppressants that act on the central nervous system. The availability of these agents differs from country to country, and any physician planning to use them should be familiar with the local regulations. Most of the drugs on the market were reviewed and approved more than 20 years ago, and are approved for short-term use only. The basis for the short-term use is two-fold. First, almost all the studies of these agents are short term. Second, the regulatory agencies are concerned about the potential for abuse, and thus have restricted all but one of the drugs to prescription use with limitations. The recent withdrawal of fenfluramine and dexfenfluramine because of concerns about their role in the development of valvular heart disease further compounds the concern of health authorities about the safety of these drugs. Because of the regulatory limitations and the lack of longer-term data on safety and efficacy, the use of the drugs approved for short-term treatment must be carefully justified. They may be useful in initiating treatment and in helping a patient who is relapsing.

Table 10: Therapeutic Strategies, Age 11-50

Age	Predictors of Overweight	Preoverweight at Risk
11-50	Positive family history of diabetes or obesity Endocrine disorders (PCO) Multiple pregnancies Marriage Smoking cessation Medication	Reduce sedentary lifestyle Low-fat/low-energy-dense diet Portion control

Sibutramine (Meridia®) is the only drug approved in the United States for long-term use, meaning up to 1 year (since that is the length of the available data). The evidence shows that weight loss of 10% or more can be produced with this drug. The side effect profile includes dry mouth, asthenia, insomnia, and constipation. It also produces a small increase in heart rate, between 2 and 5 beats a minute, and a small rise in blood pressure, between 2 and 4 mm Hg. Clinical data show no evidence of valvulopathy. Blood pressure should be followed carefully, and the drug may be inappropriate in patients with stroke, congestive heart failure, or recent myocardial infarction. It should not be used with other serotonergic drugs or drugs that inhibit monoamine oxidase.

Orlistat (Xenical®), a drug that blocks intestinal lipase, has been approved for marketing in Europe, and has received an "approvable" letter from the FDA in the United States. In clinical trials lasting up to 2 years, orlistat was associated with a mean weight loss of up to

Therapeutic Strategies

Preclinical Overweight	Clinical Overweight
Behavior therapy	Treat comorbidities
Low-fat/low-energy-dense diet	Drug treatment for overweight
Reduce sedentary lifestyle	Reduce sedentary lifestyle
	Low-fat/low-energy-dense diet
	Behavior therapy
	Surgery

10% at the end of 1 year in patients who were prescribed a 30% fat diet. As might be expected, because the drug blocks pancreatic lipase in the intestine, fecal fat loss is increased. Major side effects reported early were markedly reduced over time, implying that patients learned to use the drug effectively in relation to dietary intake of fat. The effective use of this medication requires that physicians and their staffs provide good dietary control counseling to patients.

Age Over 51

Table 11 shows the proposed treatments for this age group. By age 51, almost all of the people who become overweight have done so. Thus, preventive strategies are no longer important, and the focus is on treatment for those who are overweight or obese. The basic treatments and treatment considerations are similar to those of the younger group. However, in this age group, the argument may be stronger for directly treating comorbidities

Table 11: Therapeutic Strategies for Ages Over 51

Age	Predictors of Overweight	Preoverweight at Risk
51-75	Menopause Declining growth hormone Declining testosterone Smoking cessation Medication	Few individuals remain in this subgroup

and paying less attention to treating the clinically overweight by weight loss. For patients in this group who wish to lose weight, however, the considerations for patients between age 11 and 50 still apply. Surgery should only be considered for individuals with class II or III obesity, or who are severely overweight. This form of treatment requires skilled surgical intervention, and should only be carried out in a few places.

Criteria for Evaluating Outcomes
Criteria for Weight Loss

Figure 10 is a model of the natural history of weight change and potential criteria for success.[21] Weight rises slowly but inexorably in most of the population. The principal preventive strategy is to stop further weight gain. This alone would dramatically reduce the ravages of weight gain and prevents progression of the epidemic of obesity. A weight loss of less than 5% is unsatisfactory

Therapeutic Strategies

Preclinical Overweight
Behavior therapy
Low-fat/low-energy-
dense diet
Reduce sedentary
lifestyle

Clinical Overweight
Treat comorbidities
Drug treatment for
overweight
Reduce sedentary
lifestyle
Low-fat/low-energy-
dense diet
Behavior therapy
Surgery

for any active treatment program for overweight. Several levels of efficacy are shown, ranging from adequate to ideal. Before initiating treatment, a review of likely outcome is appropriate. An ideal outcome is a return of body weight to the normal range with no weight gain thereafter (see above).

Quality of Life
Quality of life is important for all patients. This has effects in many areas. From the health-care perspective, a reduction in comorbidities is a significant improvement. Remission of NIDDM or hypertension can reduce costs of treating these conditions, as well as delay or prevent the development of disease. Weight loss can reduce the wear and tear on joints and slow the development of osteoarthritis. Sleep apnea usually resolves.

Psychosocial improvement is greatly important to patients. Studies of patients who achieved long-term weight loss from surgical intervention (Chapter 10) comment on the improved social and economic function of previously disabled overweight patients.

Loss of 5% or more of initial weight almost always translates into improved mobility, improvement in sleep disturbances, increased exercise tolerance, and heightened self-esteem. A focus on these, rather than cosmetic outcomes, is essential.

Conclusion

Weight gain as fat results from a discrepancy between energy intake and energy expenditure (Chapter 2). The treatments outlined in chapters 6 to 10 can be related to this energy balance, as shown in Figure 10. This approach is used in the following chapters. Chapter 6 outlines behavior approaches for overweight patients. Chapters 7 and 8 address diet and exercise, the other two cornerstones for treatment of overweight. Chapter 9 covers the use of drugs in treating these patients, and Chapter 10 addresses surgery.

References

1.   Institute of Medicine: Thomas P, ed. *Weighing the Options.* Washington, DC, National Academy Press, 1995.

2.   Epstein LH, Valoski A, Wing RR, et al: Ten-year follow-up of behavioral, family-based treatment for obese children. *JAMA* 1990;264:2519-2523.

3.   Pories WJ, MacDonald KG Jr, Morgan EJ, et al: Surgical treatment of obesity and its effect on diabetes: 10-y follow-up. *Am J Clin Nutr* 1992;55:582S-585S.

4.   Bjorvell H, Rossner S: A ten-year follow-up of weight change in severely obese subjects treated in a combined behavioural modification programme. *Int J Obes Relat Metab Disord* 1992;16:623-625.

5.   Weintraub M, Sundaresan PR, Madan M, et al: Long-term weight control study. I (weeks 0 to 34). The enhancement of behavior modification, caloric restriction, and exercise by fenfluramine plus phentermine versus placebo. *Clin Pharmacol Ther* 1992;51:586-594.

6.   Garrow JS, Gardiner GT: Maintenance of weight loss in obese patients after jaw wiring. *Br J Med (Clin Res Ed)* 1981;282:858-860.

7.   Davis BR, Blaufox MD, Oberman A, et al: Reduction in long-term antihypertensive medication requirements. Effects of weight reduction by dietary intervention in overweight persons with mild hypertension. *Arch Intern Med* 1993;153:1773-1782.

8.   Bray GA, Bouchard C, James WP: Definitions and proposed current classification of obesity. In: Bray GA, Bouchard C, James WP, eds. *Handbook of Obesity.* New York, Marcel Dekker, 1997, pp 31-40.

9.   Bray GA: Classification and evaluation of the overweight patient. In: Bray GA, Bouchard C, James WP, eds. *Handbook of Obesity.* New York, Marcel Dekker, 1997, pp 831-854.

10.   U.S. Department of Health and Human Services: Screening for obesity. In: *Guide to Clinical Preventive Services,* 2nd ed. 1989, pp 219-229.

11.   American Obesity Association and Shape Up America!: *Guidance for Treatment of Adult Obesity.* Available at: http://www.shapeup.org/sua/bmi/guidance/ Accessed July 16, 1998.

12.   World Health Organization: *Consultation on Obesity,* June 1996.

13.   AACE/ACE Obesity Task Force: AACE/ACE position statement on the prevention, diagnosis, and treatment of obesity. *Endo Prac* 1997;3:162-208.

14.   U.S. Department of Health and Human Services: Body measurements. In: *Clinician's Handbook of Preventive Services: Put Prevention Into Family Practice.* 1994, pp 141-146.

15.   Roche A, Heymsfield SB, Lohman T: *Human Body Composition.* Champaign, IL, Human Kinetics, 1996.

16.   Flegal KM, Carroll MD, Kuczmarski RJ, et al: Overweight and obesity in the United States: prevalence and trends, 1960-1994. *Int J Obes Relat Metab Disord* 1998;22:39-47.

17.   Bray GA, Jordan HA, Sims EA: Evaluation of the obese patient. 1. An algorithm. *JAMA* 1976;235:1487-1491.

18.   Bray GA, Gray DS: Obesity. Part II—Treatment. *West J Med* 1988;149:555-571.

19.   Brownell KD: Dieting readiness. *Weight Control Digest* 1990;1:1-9.

20. Foster GD, Wadden TA, Vogt RA, et al: What is a reasonable weight loss? Patients' expectations and evaulations of obesity treatment outcomes. *J Consult Clin Psychol* 1997;65:79-85.

21. Rossner S: Factors determining the long-term outcome of obesity treatment. In: Bjorntorp P, Brodoff BN, eds. *Obesity*. Philadelphia, JB Lippincott, 1992, pp 712-719.

Chapter 6

Behavior Modification and the Overweight Patient

"Eat slowly: Only men in rags
And gluttons old in sin
Mistake themselves for carpet bags
And shovel victuals in."

— Sir Walter Raleigh

B
ehavior modification, or behavior therapy, has become standard in most treatment programs in the last 25 years.[1-5] The goals of this therapeutic strategy are to help patients or clients modify their eating habits, to increase their physical activity, and to make them more conscious of both of these activities in their lifestyle, thus helping them make healthier choices.[1-5] Behavior modification can affect both eating and physical activity, as suggested in the energy balance diagram in Figure 1.

Behavior Models

Behavior is the visible or outward evidence of often unknown internal processes. It can be modified by two broad but different strategies developed over the past 100 years. The first, *Pavlovian* or *conditioned behavior,* uses the ability of sentient organisms to change their behavior in response to the association of external stimuli with unconditioned behavior patterns. The classic example is the association to some other stimulus of an unconditioned response, eg, salivation when food is presented. A conditioned response occurs when

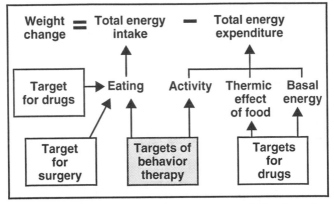

Figure 1: Behavior targets for treatment of obesity using the energy balance approach.

food is presented, along with the sound of a bell or a flashing light, in such a way that an animal or human being learns to respond to the flashing light or sound of the bell with salivation before the presentation of food. This conditioned salivary response lasts for many trials when food is not presented, but eventually is extinguished. Thus, changing association patterns is one approach to behavior change.

The second broad approach, *operant behavior*, was developed by Skinner. It enhances the likelihood of performing desired spontaneous behaviors by rewarding them. This latter approach has been most widely used in changing behavior in relation to food intake.

Behavior Programs

Behavior strategies to treat obesity, including self-monitoring of food intake, reducing environmental cues for eating, slowing the pace of eating, and increasing activities in place of eating, were initially suggested in 1962. The first successful application of these ideas was reported a few years later in a series of 8 women who lost 16 to 21 kg over 1 year. The subjects were seen individually on a schedule that was intensive in earlier phases, but decreased in intensity over time. Subjects initially were seen for 30 minutes 3 times a week for the first 4 to 5 weeks, and then biweekly for 3 months. These early results were most impressive, and behavior treatment has become significant in virtually all treatment programs. In the 1970s, a 5-kg weight loss was reproduced reliably, but 'relapse' was common. In the past decade, efforts have focused on improving the magnitude of the weight loss, improving maintenance of weight loss, and matching treatment strategies to individual patients. This involves a number of additional strategies, including partner training, training to prevent relapses, and adding anorectic drugs or very-low-calorie diets and exercise.

Table 1 summarizes the research and behavior therapy since the early papers in the 1970s through 1995.[4-6] Each period contains 5 to 17 papers; a large literature occurred in the first 15 years after introduction of this treatment. This table yields several insights. First, sample sizes gradually increase. Initial weights also increase, from a mean of 73 kg to more than 90 kg. Second, the length of treatment rises from just longer than 8 weeks to more than 20 weeks. Degree of weight loss increases with this, accounting for the improved results with longer treatment. However, rates of weight loss do not increase. Attrition with behavior therapy has been surprisingly low. Attrition in the early studies ranged from 10% to 13%, but even in larger, longer studies, it only ranged between 17% and 24%. Attrition is much higher for other treatments. Behavior treatment produces weight losses between 9% and 10%, which is very satisfactory (Figure 2). The relationship of duration of treatment to weight loss also is clear in this figure. As length of treatment increases, more weight is lost.

ABCs of Behavior Treatment

The three elements of behavior treatment for obesity are the ABCs, or the **a**ntecedents, **b**ehavior of eating, and **c**onsequences of the behavior change. Determining the

169

Table 1: Summary of Research on Behavior Therapy for Obesity (1974-1995)[4]

	1974	1978	1984
Number of studies	15	17	15
Sample size	53.1	53.1	54.0
Initial weight (kg)	73.4	87.3	88.7
Weeks of treatment	8.4	10.5	13.2
Weight loss (kg)	3.8	4.2	6.9
Loss per week (kg)	0.5	0.4	0.5
Attrition (%)	11.4	12.9	10.6
Weeks of follow-up	15.5	30.3	58.4
Loss at follow-up	4.0	4.1	4.4

BT = behavior therapy; VL = very-low-calorie diet. Behavior therapy plus very-low-calorie diet was included because much of the behavior therapy for obesity includes a very-low-calorie diet. The data, from 1974 to 1990, are taken from Wadden and VanItallie. Data are updated from 1991 to 1995. The research shown in the table pertains only to studies of behavior therapy for obesity in adults.[4-6]

antecedents to eating involves observing and recording the behaviors related to eating. This self-monitoring identifies settings of eating. It involves writing down the kinds of food eaten, the places where food is eaten, how frequently food is eaten, and the emotional setting in which it is eaten. Using these self-monitoring reports, individuals can identify possibly changeable antecedent problems related to times and places of eating. Two different approaches to self-monitoring have been employed. One uses a table in which all behaviors associated with eating are simultaneously recorded (Table 2). An alternative approach focuses on one component at a time (see Appendix B, Guide to Behavior Change Toward Better Eating). Thus, hunger, frequency of eating, place of eating, and associated activities are each analyzed separately. Expe-

1985-1987	1988-1990	1991-1995	
13	5	3	4
71.3	71.6	97.3	114.5
87.2	91.9	93.3	104.5
15.6	21.3	20.7	21.1
8.4	8.5	8.8	22.0
0.5	0.4	0.5	1.1
13.8	21.8	17.0	24.0
48.3	53.0	43.0	71.0
5.3	5.6	7.9	12.1

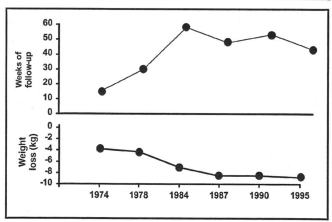

Figure 2: Summary of research on behavior therapy of obesity from 1974 to 1995.

rience suggests that focusing on behaviors one at a time is easier than all of them at once. We use the behavior approach outlined in the appendix. A useful manual of behavior strategies has been published by Brownell.[2]

The 'B' of the ABCs of behavior modification involves the behavior of eating. It uses stimulus control to break the chain of events between an antecedent for eating and the eating or behavior event itself. A number of techniques have been developed to provide stimulus control (Table 3).

Among the simplest techniques are restricting the number of eating places or the utensils used for eating. Others involve picking up a glass of water between each bite, chewing the food a defined number of times, or excusing oneself from the table for a time. The goal is to separate the events that trigger eating from the eating itself. For example, for a patient who picks up doughnuts at a doughnut shop on the way to work each morning, a stimulus control strategy would be planning a different route to work. Self-monitoring helps identify these problems and provides feedback to monitor changes. Keeping food out of sight is another technique.

The third component of classic behavior modification involves manipulating the 'C' or consequences for self-reward. Collecting points toward the reward of a new hairdo, new clothes, or other event can be an approach to rewarding good behavior. Contingency contracts, ie, payment of money for attaining certain milestones, also is widely used.

The Skinner approach offers several techniques for reinforcing good behavior. These include rewarding changes in behavior rather than rewarding weight loss. A serious error is using food as a reward for these behavior changes. Rewards should be reinforcing. Money works for almost anybody but, for women, clothing, hairstyling, or other rewards can be very effective. The reward should be received as soon as possible after the improved behavior to reinforce the value of the good behavior. Money rewards must be carefully constructed. Behavior goals must be clearly defined, and the time frame for achieving these goals must be stated. Partial changes on the way to the final target may be important to reinforce the direction of improved behavior. Goals must be realistic, and the rewards achievable. Several behavior techniques have been added to the classic approaches of the 1970s. The first involves assertiveness training, to help patients learn to say "no" and develop positive 'self-talk' by using cognitive strategies.

Social support for the individual in a behavior weight-loss program is very important. One approach to strengthening social support is the 'buddy system,' which includes a friend or family member who can provide social support and reinforcement for the positive behavior changes that the patient is attempting to implement. The buddy system requires that the buddy be sympathetic to the goals of the patient and the program. Use of partners has been suggested, and has had variable success. Sabotage by friends and relatives can particularly damage an individual in a weight-loss program. For some spouses, weight loss by their loved one can be threatening. Marriages can break up if a partner is successful in achieving significant weight loss. The possibility of sabotage requires careful evaluation at the beginning, and continued monitoring during therapy. Individuals who provide support for weight loss can be involved in two ways. In some programs, the individuals are brought in and receive some basic information about the goals and strategies of the program. Alternatively, the patient can transmit the information to a friend or colleague. Whichever is used, the buddy should provide as much social support as possible for the weight and behavior goals.

As part of the social support, providing opportunities for role playing for difficult situations is important. Parties, holidays, vacations, and the unmeaning negative input of innocent bystanders all require familiarity with techniques for refusing food when it is offered. One strategy is to help people with assertiveness training, a technique for learning how to say "no" and continuing to repeat "no" even when urged repeatedly in the opposite direction.

Table 2: Self-Monitoring Form for Recording Food Intake and Situational Factors Related to Eating

List each food item and describe method of preparation (eg, baked, fried, boiled, broiled, raw).

Food item/ Beverage	Quantity	Time of Day	Duration of Eating	Meal/ Snack	

These important strategies can be practiced with a partner or within group settings as part of the learning procedures for changing behaviors and their consequences.

Another new component to behavior therapy involves internal or cognitive self-support. Everybody has continu-

Level of Hunger 0 = none 3 = extreme hunger	Activity During Eating	Location of Eating	Social Situation (Family Meal, Eating Out, Meal at Work, Alone)	Feeling/Mood Before Eating	After Eating

ously running internal conversations. These can be positive or negative. For example, a patient who eats a piece of cake that is not on the 'diet' has at least two ways to respond. First, the internal response could be, "Oh, you idiot, you've blown your diet." As a consequence, the patient may

Table 3: Stimulus Control Techniques

- Eat three meals a day.
- Eat approximately the same time each day.
- Eat as many meals as possible in the same place in the house.
- Eat while seated at a table.
- Focus on food.
- Eliminate distractions such as reading or watching television.
- Use small plates for food. Do not put food containers on the table.
- Cook only small amounts of food. Slow pace of eating by putting down utensils between bites, or taking a drink of water.
- Put foods in open rather than transparent containers.
- Do not use high-calorie condiments. Shop shortly after eating to reduce likelihood of purchasing high-energy preferred foods.
- Clean plates directly into the garbage.
- Avoid second servings.

eat the whole cake. An alternative internal conversation is "I ate cake when it wasn't in my plan, but now I can do something to modify my plan to get back on track." This positive problem-solving approach is much more likely than negative self-deprecatory comments to be successful.

All successful programs also include some component of stress management. Stress is part of everyday life at home and work. One consequence of these stressful situations can be uncontrolled eating. Strategies that reduce individuals' choice of foods when confronted with stress can be very helpful. One good approach is to help people identify a relaxing place that, with the eyes shut and a few deep breaths, allows the stress to subside. This technique can greatly reduce tension and stress. If such stress reduction does not occur, food intake for susceptible individuals may be an unwanted consequence.

Results of Behavior Therapy

The literature on behavior therapy for obesity is extensive (Table 1). Several illustrations emphasize the importance of this procedure for many overweight patients.

The impact in children is most striking.[6] Using behavior therapy, children and one or both parents, compared with the child alone or a limited-treatment control group, showed dramatic 10-year results (Figure 3). All three groups initially lost a significant amount of weight. However, children treated with their parents maintained less excess weight over the next 10 years.[6] Because children ages 3 to 10 with one overweight parent are highly unlikely to remain overweight as young adults (Chapter 4), these techniques are desirable for this group.

Another 10-year study from Sweden is presented in Figure 4.[7] The initial program compared weight loss in patients with their jaws wired together, with a vigorous behavior therapy program that included periodic hospitalization, if needed. An observational control group lost no weight. The jaw-wired patients lost most weight initially; however, after the jaw wires were removed and behavior therapy substituted, they ended up with the same weight loss as patients who only had behavior therapy. Results from the behavior group are shown in Figure 4. During active treatment in the first year, women lost nearly 15 kg. Using booster sessions and other techniques for up to 4 years, most weight loss was maintained in those who continued the program, even when followed for 10 years.

Because weight changes of more than 5% to 10% are considered successful (Chapter 5), realistic rewards should occur at steps along the way. Instead of setting goals for weight loss of 20% or more, which cannot be achieved by

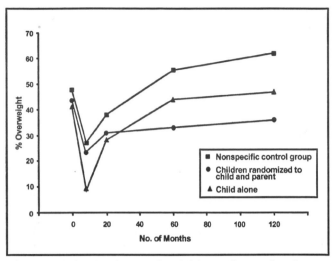

Figure 3: Behavior therapy for children. The results of treating a child with parent(s), treating the child alone, and a nonspecific control group are shown at intervals to 10 years.[6]

the usual techniques and produce disappointed doctors and patients, more realistic goals should be set. In a 1-year follow-up of 590 patients treated with behavior therapy, weight loss averaged 5.8 kg (12.8 lb).[8] Of these 590 individuals, 17.5% were either at or above their entry weight 1 year later. At follow-up 5 years later, the mean weight loss of 426 patients at the end of treatment was 6.9 kg (15.1 lb) in 116 men, and 4.2 kg (9.3 lb) in 310 women. At the 1-year follow-up in this group, weight loss was 7.4 kg for the men and 5.4 kg for the women. At 5 years, weight loss was 6.3 kg below baseline for the men and 4.3 kg for the women, indicating that 50% maintained or continued to lose weight. This is encouraging for people beginning a behavior weight-loss program.

Because behavior therapy does not cure obesity, much effort has recently focused on secondary prevention of weight regain. One group of studies showing the effect of

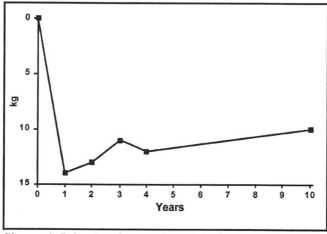

Figure 4: *Behavior therapy for adults.* [7]

adding extra support is presented in Figure 5. Note that behavior therapy alone produced a weight loss of more than 10 kg, but regain was evident in all groups at 18 months. Additional weight loss occurred with each additional therapeutic element. The largest weight loss and least regain were observed when exercise, social contact, and therapist contact all were used (Figure 5).[3] Thus, behavior therapy can be effective when properly used.

In addition to the items above, several lessons can be drawn from the behavior literature.[9] In a retrospective review, several behavior techniques proved more useful than others (Table 4). Self-monitoring heads the list. Records of food eaten and associated activities can be a constant reminder of problem areas. Stimulus control strategies (breaking the chain of causes for eating) was second. This can result from the self-monitoring that provides clues for needed changes. The other three—stress management, cognitive strategies, and contingency management—reflect greater self-awareness of eating and how to control events surrounding food intake.

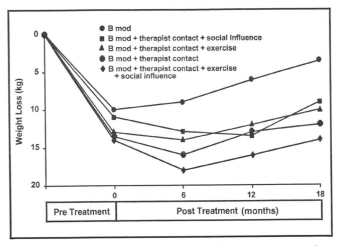

Figure 5: Effect on weight loss of adding support to a basic behavior program.[3] B mod=behavior modification.

Several behavior and lifestyle changes predict successful behavior weight loss[9] (Table 5). People with positive feelings about themselves and others have a strong sense of well-being. This can be one result of increased activity. People who believe they are losing weight for themselves, rather than for others, are internally motivated. They perceive that they are in control, which is a good predictor of success. This is associated with the next item, a focus on positive changes in health, fitness, and appearance. A social support system surrounding the patient that focuses on health, not weight, is another predictor of success. This helps support the patient's goals and aspirations. Other predictors of successful weight-loss maintenance are increased physical activity and reduction of dietary fat.

Predictors of failure include negative feelings, depression, anxiety, and anger. Individuals who are continually tested by travel, entertaining, and eating away from home

Table 4: Most Helpful Behavior Techniques

- Self-monitoring
- Stimulus control
- Stress management
- Cognitive behavior strategies
- Contingency management

Table 5: Behavior Predictors of Successful Weight Loss

- Positive feelings
- Internal motivation
- Focusing on positive changes in health, fitness, and appearance
- Social support

find it more difficult to control food intake and physical activity, and are more likely to fail. Patients who test themselves by seeing what they can get away with are also likely to fail because they are likely to try food in this context, with bad results.

Work-Site Programs

In addition to the classic techniques of individual or group behavior therapy, other strategies have been used to broaden the reach of these techniques.[10] Stunkard and Brownell have used the work site to apply behavior modification to the treatment of obesity. Attrition was a significant problem, as in most outpatient treatment programs. Interestingly, however, the drop-out rate was lower in groups, and weight loss was 3.6 kg in those completing a 16-week program.

Table 6: Information About Behavior Resources for Weight Loss

National Community-Based
Multicenter Weight Loss Programs

Diet Center Inc.
921 Penn Ave.
Pittsburgh, PA 15222
412/338-8700

Nutrition Counseling	Individual counseling.
Behavior Counseling	Individual and group classes.
Activity Plan	Individualized exercise goals developed by counselor with use of computer program.
Food Plan	Emphasizes real food available in grocery stores. Foods that meet Diet Center nutritional criteria are sold in centers.
Adult Calorie Levels	Men: 1,300 base Women: 945 base Additional calories at the counselor's discretion. Some centers customize calorie intake based on body composition analysis.

Diet Composition
- Protein: 16%-27%
- Fat: 20%-28%
- Carbohydrate: 52%-62%
- Nutrient levels depend on program phase.

Contact Frequency	Recommended daily during reducing phase; throughout stabilization phase 3: 3 days/week; maintenance once a week for 1 year
Maintenance	1-year plan.
Cost	Average full-service program for 30-lb weight loss and maintenance: $600. Cost varies by location and center.
Staff Training	Certification training at corporate office and continuous seminars in the field; 1,500 centers in the United States and Canada.

Jenny Craig, Inc.
445 Marine View Drive, Suite 300
Del Mar, CA 92014
619/259-7000

Nutrition Counseling	Individual counseling.
Behavior Counseling	Group class discussions assisted by videotapes. Audio tapes available at additional cost.
Activity Plan	Personal Exercise Plan booklet; walking program booklet with two videotapes and two audio tapes.
Food Plan	Proprietary food line with weekly preplanned menus, plus fresh fruits, vegetables, grains, and milk products.
Adult Calorie Levels	Men: 1,200-1,700 Women: 1,000-1,500

(continued on next page)

Table 6: Information About Behavior Resources for Weight Loss *(continued)*

Diet Composition
- Protein: 20%
- Fat: 20%
- Carbohydrate: 60%

Contact Frequency	Twice weekly: (1) 20-minute individual consultation and (1) 40-minute class.
Maintenance	1-year plan; 50% refund with maintenance of reduced weight for 1 year.
Cost	Average full-service program for all the weight one wants to lose, including maintenance, $178. Food costs $10/d.
Staff Training	40-hour training program with 8-hour follow-up and individual training in center; 520 centers in the United States and Canada.

Nutri/System, Inc.
380 Sentry Pkwy.
Blue Bell, PA 19422
215/940-3000

Nutrition Counseling	Individual counseling.
Behavior Counseling	Small-group classes tailored to the individual through use of a behavior profile.
Activity Plan	3-part personalized activity plan for daily activities, walking, low-intensity stretching, and aerobics. Two videotapes of graduated aerobic activity in conjunction with the Aerobic and Fitness Association of America.

Food Plan	Proprietary food line providing individual client selection from nearly 100 items. Fresh fruits, vegetables, and nonfat milk from grocery store.
Adult Calorie Levels	Men: 1,200-1,500 or higher, depending on individual needs. Women: 1,000-1,500 or higher, depending on individual needs. (Canada: 1,200 calories)

Diet Composition
- Protein: 22%-23% (Canada: 26%)
- Fat: 15%-16% (Canada: 18%)
- Carbohydrate: 62% (Canada: 56%)

Contact Frequency	Once weekly for 1 hour, and Care Calls by phone. Clients may visit center additional times if desired.
Maintenance	1-year personalized plan; 50% refund with maintenance of reduced weight for 1 year.
Cost	Average full-service program for 30-lb weight loss and maintenance, $300-$400. Food costs $9.50 a day.
Staff Training	Nutri/System formal classroom and in-center training and certification for nutrition and behavior counselors. Counselors continue to receive individual training after certification. Approximately 1,800 centers in the United States and Canada.

(continued on next page)

Table 6: Information About Behavior Resources for Weight Loss *(continued)*

Weight Watchers International Inc.
Jericho Atrium
500 N. Broadway
Jericho, NY 11753-2196
516/939-0400

Nutrition and Behavior Counseling	Group meetings (25-30 average) providing: specific instructions on how to follow the program; support for meeting weight loss challenges; motivation to encourage program adherence; and leader who has successfully completed program as 'role model.'
Activity Plan	Individualized, multilevel exercise plan emphasizing low-intensity, long-duration aerobic activities. Includes guidelines for toning and stretching.
Food Plan	Based on set number of selections from each of six food lists using foods sold in grocery stores.
Adult Calorie Levels	Men: 1,200-1,600 Women: 1,000-1,450

Diet Composition
- Protein: 12%-20%
- Fat: <30%
- Carbohydrate: 50%-60%

Contact Frequency	Once weekly for up to 1 hour.
Maintenance	Individualized maintenance plans plus lifetime membership available at no cost if reduced weight is maintained.

Cost Registration fee (average $75) and weekly group meeting charges (average $10/week). Approximately $175 for 30-lb weight loss, based on a maximum of 1 to 2 lb/week. Discounts available for prepayment.

Staff Training Company-trained 'graduates' formerly on program, must maintain weight. Initial: 30 hours classroom plus exam; 30 hours 'in-meeting' coaching. On-going: 2 hours every 6 weeks; annual reassessment of skills and program knowledge; 20,000 meetings in 5,000 locations in the United States and Canada.

Self-Help Groups

Overeaters Anonymous
World Service Office
P.O. Box 92870
Los Angeles, CA 90009
213/542-8363

Nutrition and Behavior Counseling Nonprofit support group. Members participate in weekly meetings, retreats, and annual conventions. Follows Alcoholics Anonymous 12-step program to correct behavior. No food plans, nutrition counseling, or exercise component. Encourages members who seek such counseling to consult qualified professionals.

Activity Plan None

(continued on next page)

Table 6: Information About Behavior Resources for Weight Loss *(continued)*

Food Plan	None
Contact Frequency	Weekly meetings.
Cost	No membership fees.
Staff Training	Members (nonprofessional) conduct activities; no training required; 11,000 groups worldwide.

TOPS Club, Inc.
(Take Off Pounds Sensibly)
P.O. Box 07360
Milwaukee, WI 53207
800/932-8677

Nutrition Counseling	Members referred to their private physicians for diets and counseling.
Behavior Counseling	None
Activity Plan	None

Self-Help Programs

A number of self-help groups for weight control now exist in the United States and other countries. Among these are noncommercial groups such as Overeaters Anonymous and Take Off Pounds Sensibly (TOPS), and commercial groups such as Weight Watchers International, Diet Center Inc., Jenny Craig, and Nutri/System (Table 6). Studies on these groups and their effectiveness are limited, but attrition clearly is a problem. One study of TOPS evaluated 350,000 members in 12,000 chapters. Almost all were females. Among the features

Food Plan	Exchange food lists.
Adult Calorie Levels	1,200-1,800; specific food plan
Diet Composition	
• Protein: 20%-22%	
• Fat: 35%-38%	
• Carbohydrate: 40%-44%	
• Recommended but not required.	
Contact Frequency	Weekly in local chapters.
Maintenance	Members graduate to KOPS (Keep Off Pounds Sensibly), an inner honor society that further motivates them to maintain new weights.
Cost	$16/year
Staff Training	Volunteer chapter leaders receive guidance from area TOPS coordinators; 11,650 chapters worldwide.

of the weekly meeting were the official weigh-in and announcement of individual changes in weight. In studying 21 chapters in the Philadelphia area, Garb and Stunkard noted that the mean weight loss was 6.8 kg (15 lb) ± 6.8 kg.[11] When the same chapters were reviewed 2 years later, mean weight loss was 6.4 kg (14 lb) ± 7.7 kg (17 lb). The rate of attrition in TOPS and several other groups ranged from 40% to more than 70%. Half the clients stopped attending after 10 to 50 weeks. In a comprehensive survey of weight loss in Weight Watchers groups, Ashwell and Garrow noted that patients in the United Kingdom lost an average 11.8 kg (26 lb) in 30 weeks.[12] Attrition includes those who successfully achieve their weight goal and those who do not. The data do not allow for distinction between them.

Psychoanalysis

Psychoanalysis also has been used for the treatment of obesity. In a retrospective study, 72 psychoanalysts collected information on 84 obese patients and a control sample of 63 normal-weight patients.[13] Although obesity was the chief complaint for only 6 of these patients, weight loss at 42 months of psychoanalytic treatment compared favorably with those after traditional medical efforts. Of those obese patients receiving psychoanalysis, 47% lost more than 9 kg and 19% lost more than 18 kg. The percentage of obese patients suffering from disparagement of body image also significantly decreased. This decline, from 40% to 14%, is an unexpectedly good result for this chronic and intractable disorder. Thus, behavior treatments ranging from psychoanalysis to work sites, and from family and couples training to self-help groups, offer significant contributions to short- and long-term effectiveness in treating obesity.

References

1.   Brownell KD: Dieting readiness. *Weight Control Digest* 1990;1:1-10.

2.   Brownell KD: *The LEARN Program for Weight Control.* Dallas, American Health Publishing, 1992.

3.   Perri MG, Nezu AM, Viegener BJ: *Improving the Long-Term Management of Obesity: Theory, Research and Clinical Guidelines.* New York, John Wiley, 1992.

4.   Williamson DA, Perrin LA: Behavioral therapy for obesity. *Endocrinol Metab Clin North Am* 1996;25:943-954.

5.   Wing RR: Behavioral approaches to the treatment of obesity. In: Bray GA, Bouchard C, James WP, eds. *Handbook of Obesity.* New York, Marcel Dekker, 1997, pp 855-873.

6.   Epstein LH, Valoski A, Wing RR, et al: Ten-year follow-up of behavioral, family-based treatment for obese children. *JAMA* 1990;264:2519-2523.

7.   Bjorvell H, Rossner S: A ten-year follow-up of weight change in severely obese subjects treated in a combined behavioural modification programme. *Int J Obes Relat Metab Disord* 1992;16:623-625.

8.   Kramer FM, Jeffery RW, Forster JL, et al: Long-term follow-up of behavioral treatment for obesity: patterns of weight regain among men and women. *Int J Obes* 1989;13:123-126.

9.   Foreyt JP: Factors common to successful therapy for the obese patient. *Med Sci Sports Exerc* 1991;23:292-297.

10.   Stunkard AJ, Brownell KD: Work-site treatment for obesity. *Am J Psychiatry* 1980;137:252-253.

11.   Garb JR, Stunkard AJ: Effectiveness of a self-help group in obesity control. A further assessment. *Arch Intern Med* 1974;134:716-720.

12.   Ashwell M, Garrow JS: A survey of three slimming and weight control organizations in the U.K. *Nutrition* 1975;29:347-356.

13.   Rand C, Stunkard AJ: Obesity and psychoanalysis. *Am J Psychiatry* 1978;135:547-551.

Chapter 7

Nutrition, Diet, and Treatment of Overweight

"Let me have men about me that are fat;
Sleek-headed men, and such as sleep o'night
Yond Cassius has a lean and hungry look:
He thinks too much; such men are dangerous.
— Shakespeare
Julius Caesar
Act I, Scene 2

Diet springs eternal in the hearts of the overweight; a renewal of interest peaks each year in late winter.[1,2] For nearly 150 years, numerous diets have been extolled for their benefits in the treatment and prevention of obesity. The effects of diet composition during weight gain, in which the composition of the diet may be greatly important, must be distinguished from the composition of the diet during weight loss, in which no evidence suggests that modifying the composition of the diet has any differential effect as long as the total energy value of the diet is less than that required for energy maintenance.

Dietary approaches ranging from starvation with no available calories, to very-low-energy diets and low-energy diets varying in composition, all have been recommended (Table 1). Long-term starvation without careful supervision is hazardous and is not recommended. Although, in principle, a very-low-energy diet of 400 kcal/d

Table 1: Classification of Diets

Type of Diet	Energy Value (kcal/d)
Starvation	0-200
Very-Low-Calorie	200-800
• Optifast®	
• Medifast®	
• Modifast®	
Low-Calorie	>800
• Balanced-deficit	
• Low-fat/high-carbohydrate	
• High-protein	
• Portion-controlled	

should produce more weight loss than a very-low-energy diet of 800 kcal/d, this has not occurred in practice. Because a larger variety of nutrients are available with a higher energy level, we believe that a very-low-energy diet with less than 800 kcal/d is unnecessary and undesirable as a treatment for obesity. For weight maintenance and prevention of weight gain, a low-fat diet appears to be the diet of choice.

The long-term success of all diets is low because people stop following the diet—they become noncompliant. However, some people clearly maintain long-term weight loss by following a new eating plan. This difference is attributable to one of several factors. First, evidence clearly suggests that successful weight losers are people who modify their dietary eating patterns to consume less fat.[3] Second, this altered dietary pattern requires motivation, which is a major requirement of any successful therapeutic program. Loss of motivation and failure to continue the dietary changes necessary to consume less fat and fewer calories are followed by weight regain.

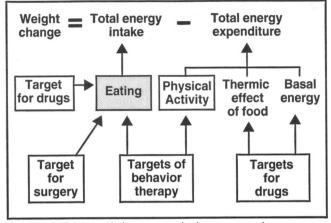

Figure 1: Diet and the energy balance equation.

Dietary Approaches to Obesity

This chapter describes the techniques for modifying food intake to achieve weight loss. Figure 1 uses the energy balance diagram to show where diets work (by reducing food intake).

The popularity of diets resembles that of fashion; diets come and go. Table 1 lists some diets, which can be divided into several groups based on relative energy level, whether they use natural foods or formulas, and the nature of the foods that are emphasized. This chapter examines energy and nutrient requirements, and then evaluates specific diets. Table 2 lists some programs and informational services to help plan and carry out a diet.

Energy and Nutrient Requirements

Maintenance of stable energy stores requires that the energy in the food be balanced by complete oxidation (Chapter 2). While eating, individuals are in positive energy balance, and between meals they are in negative energy balance. Homeothermic animals, like human beings, maintain a constant body temperature as well as a stable internal milieu for muscular movement for heartbeat and other needs. Over 24 hours, individuals are in either slightly positive or slightly negative energy balance. Weight maintenance requires the patient to keep these deviations small, with an average value of zero over weeks to months. The basic requirement for weight loss is to hold a negative energy balance for most days.

Energy Needs

The first information needed to develop a dietary plan is some idea of the patient's energy requirement. This can be done by one of two methods: (1) measuring resting energy expenditure using a ventilated hood or respiration calorimeter; or (2) estimating energy expenditure from formulas.[4-7]

Resting Metabolic Rate

The best direct method for assessing energy needs is measurement of resting metabolic rate corrected for the individual's level of activity. Although total energy expenditure can be estimated in a variety of ways, including doubly labeled water, heart rate, and various activity monitors, the most practical way is to measure resting metabolic rate with a ventilated hood system. The resting metabolic rate is then multiplied by an activity factor between 1.3 for very sedentary people to 1.7 for the highest levels of activity, to obtain an estimate of 24-hour energy expenditure.

Formulas for Estimating Energy Expenditure

The second method is to use nomograms or formulas to estimate energy expenditure. A food nomogram developed by the Mayo Clinic is shown in Figure 2.[6] Starting with body weight and height, surface area is determined. Using age, basal metabolism is determined and, with an estimate of activity factor, daily food allowance then is estimated. The second approach is to use the formulas in Table 3 from the World Health Organization.[7] A simple rule of thumb also can be used; overweight

Table 2: Behavior Resources for Weight Loss

Registered Dietitians

Registered dietitians in private practice, hospital-based programs, public health clinics, or other outpatient settings

Nutrition Counseling	Individual or group counseling.
Behavior Counseling	Individual or group counseling depending on individual needs. Variety of counseling strategies.
Activity Plan	Individual guidance and support.
Food Plan	Based on individual eating plan. Considers ethnic, social, and financial factors.
Adult Calorie Levels	Depend on weight loss goals and medical conditions. Calorie range varies from low to moderate intake with increased activity.
Diet Composition	Individualized
Contact Frequency	Based on need and goals. Direct contact and phone follow-up included. Varies: once a week to bimonthly, then quarterly and biyearly. Intensive intervention initially. Medical visits and laboratory tests as required.
Maintenance	Considered critical. Yearly plan available.
Cost	Varies with services needed.
Staff Training	Strong science and nutrition background with a minimum of bachelor's

degree and advanced training. Must meet continuing education requirements to maintain registration. In addition to or as part of private practice, may be associated with physicians, psychologists, or exercise physiologists.

Very-Low-Calorie Medically Supervised Hospital- or Office-Based Plans

Optifast
Novartis Nutrition Corp.
5320 W. 23rd St.
P.O. Box 370
Minneapolis, MN 55440
612/925-2100

Nutrition and Behavior Counseling Medically supervised, hospital-based program using a very-low-calorie diet. Behavior modification, psychologic group support, nutrition education, exercise, and medical monitoring (physician visits, laboratory testing) weekly for 26 weeks.

Adult Calorie Levels Very-low-calorie diet (VLCD) phase (12 weeks): patients consume liquid supplement (Optifast 700 or 800) 5 times daily, providing approximately 420 to 800 calories. Refeeding phase (6 weeks): reintroduction of solid food, with gradual increase in calories. Stabilization phase (7 weeks): approximately 1,200-1,500-calorie stabilization diet, supplement discontinued.

(continued on next page)

Table 2: Behavior Resources for Weight Loss
(continued)

Diet Composition
- Protein: 35%-67%
- Fat: 4%-15%
- Carbohydrate: 29%-50%

Contact Frequency	Weekly clinic visits with behaviorist and dietitian. Weekly physician visits during VLCD phase; biweekly thereafter.
Maintenance	Stabilization phase plus 26-week Encore Program, a behavior-based maintenance program including exercise, nutrition education, and group, with the physician available as needed.
Cost	Varies among centers; approximately $3,000 for 2-week program. Encore maintenance program approximately $500.
Staff Training	Registered dietitians and nurses, physicians, exercise specialists, and psychologists. One-week intensive training offered at least six times a year; 3-day annual postgraduate advanced training; 12-volume program manual.

(Other national, hospital-based programs such as New Direction [Ross Laboratories] and Health Management Resources are similar approaches.)

patients require approximately 10 kcal/lb of body weight, or 22 kcal/kg. Thus, a 100-kg (220-lb) individual requires approximately 2,200 kcal/d for weight maintenance. This number is a little higher for young individuals, but serves as an easy guideline for energy needs.

Medifast
Jason Pharmaceuticals, Inc.
P.O. Box 370
Owing Mills, MD 21117
301/581-8042

Activity Plan Education component is the Lifestyles Program. Group sessions or individual counseling. Patient material is a 16-chapter guide. Group leader's manual has a corresponding lesson plan. The 16 chapters cover nutrition, behavior changes, and exercise.

Adult Calorie Levels 16-week fasting phase; 4-6 week re-feeding phase; optional 12-week stabilization phase. High-protein, low-carbohydrate formula. Three formulas, two protocols. Medifast 55 or 70 intake is 5 packets/day (440-480 calories), no food. Alternate plan adds minimal (600-650 calories). Medifast Plus: 880-calorie daily intake—4 packets (375 calories) and a defined meal (505 calories).

(continued on next page)

A reduction in caloric intake of 500 kcal/d below requirements translates into a weight loss of about 0.5 kg (1 lb) a week if the diet is followed carefully. A 220-lb (100-kg) individual needs about 2,200 kcal/d. A 500-kcal deficit provides 1,700 kcal/d, leading to a theoreti-

Table 2: Behavior Resources for Weight Loss
(continued)

Diet Composition
- Protein: 43%-53%
- Fat: 2%-25%
- Carbohydrate: 28%-35%

Contact Frequency	Once weekly for medical check and counseling. Physician visit required twice a month.
Maintenance	Lifestyles II is a 24-week group program. Group Leader's Manual gives lesson plans, patient activity sheets, and handout copies.
Cost	Varies by location and extent of program. Average cost is $65-$75/week for office visit and supplement; 16-week program $1,040-$1,200. Lifestyles II 24-week maintenance program, $192-$288.
Staff Training	Three-volume program manuals supplied to associate physicians. One-day training course covering program and patient management; 24 training sessions offered nationwide for physicians and staff. Annual 2-day obesity education seminar.

cal 3,500-kcal deficit each week until a new plateau is reached, about 170 lb (80 kg). An alternative is to provide diets with fixed energy levels. Common levels are 1,200

Meal Replacements

Ultra-Slim-Fast & Slim-Fast
Slim-Fast Foods Co.
777 South Flagler Drive
West Tower, Suite 1400
West Palm Beach, FL 33401
561/833-9920

Nutrition and Behavior Counseling	Self-motivated, self-monitored program. Consumer brochures available on meal planning, shopping, and dining out.
Activity Plan:	Product insert suggests 30 minutes of brisk walking, 3 times a week at minimum.
Food Plan:	Ultra Slim-Fast shakes for breakfast and lunch; 2-3 snacks up to 250 calories, and 600-calorie dinner of solid food.
Adult Calorie Levels	200/serving

Diet Composition
- Protein: 31%
- Fat: 6%
- Carbohydrate: 63%
- (with 8 oz skim milk)

(continued on next page)

kcal/d for women and 1,500 kcal/d for men, reflecting gender differences in body composition and energy expenditure, but not considering differences in body weight.

Table 2: Behavior Resources for Weight Loss
(continued)

Maintenance	Ultra Slim-Fast shake for breakfast; low-fat meals for lunch and dinner. Regular exercise recommended.
Cost	Powdered shake mix: <$1.00/serving when mixed with milk. Cost of solid food meal additional.

DynaTrim
Wyeth-Ayerst Laboratories
P.O. Box 8299
Philadelphia, PA 19101
610/902-1200

Nutrition and Behavior Counseling	Self-motivated, self-monitored program. Consumer brochure available.
Activity Plan	Product literature suggests exercise, particularly walking; also provides tips for behavior modification.
Food Plan	DynaTrim shake or mousse for breakfast, lunch, and snack; solid food meal for dinner.

Effect of Diet Composition
on Weight Loss and Weight Maintenance

Initial weight loss on any hypocaloric diet is more rapid than subsequent weight loss. This occurs for three reasons. First, glycogen stores and the associated intracellular water are rapidly mobilized to provide glucose for the brain and nerves. As this glucose is used up over 24 to 72 hours, gluconeogenesis accelerates and the rate of weight loss slows to a steady rate. With a fixed, lower-

Adult Calorie Levels 220/serving

Diet Composition
- Protein: 31%
- Fat: 13%
- Carbohydrate: 56%
- (with 8 oz 1%-fat milk)

Maintenance	DynaTrim once or twice daily to replace a meal or as a snack; low-calorie meals. Menu guide provided with examples of balanced lunches and dinners.
Cost	Powdered shake mix: $.75/serving when mixed with milk. Cost of solid food meal additional.

(Use of liquid meal replacements for self-devised very-low-calorie-diet plans is not recommended.)

energy diet, variations of fat, carbohydrate, and protein levels do not affect the rate of weight loss over 60 to 90 days. Second, energy needs gradually fall as weight is lost because less energy is required to move a lighter body. Third, energy requirements adapt, reducing the response to a hypocaloric diet.

Diet composition is an important difference in weight maintenance and weight gain. To maintain energy stores, the amount of dietary fat and carbohydrate must equal

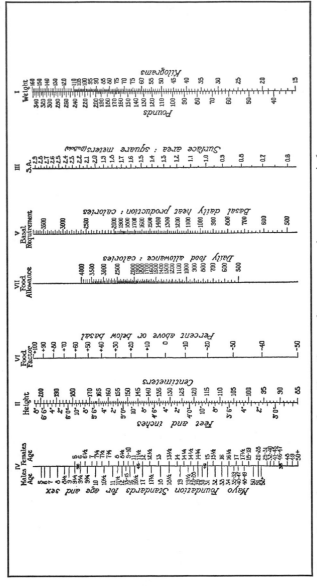

Figure 2: Food nomogram for estimating surface area and energy needs.[6]

204

the amount of fat and carbohydrate oxidized for energy purposes. Because it may be difficult to reduce carbohydrate oxidation on a high-fat, low-carbohydrate diet, a low-fat, high-carbohydrate diet is generally preferable during weight maintenance. Indeed, success in maintaining weight loss is related to whether patients modify their long-term dietary patterns to maintain this lower fat intake. One study compared a low-fat ad-lib diet with a fixed-energy diet in a group of patients who were randomly assigned to the diets after an initial weight-loss program, in which they lost, on average, slightly more than 13 kg. At 1 and 2 years after beginning the diets, the patients assigned to the low-fat ad-lib diet were significantly lighter, although both groups had regained some weight.[8]

Nutritional Considerations

Planning a low-energy diet involves several nutritional considerations. What foods should constitute this diet? Should these foods be chosen by the patient or provided in portion-controlled form?[4,9,10]

Food contains more than 40 nutrients, which are needed in proper amounts for all bodily functions. The macronutrients consist of water, oxygen, protein, carbohydrate, and fat, while the micronutrients consist of all additional vitamins and minerals (Chapter 1). Table 4 lists Recommended Dietary Intakes published by the National Research Council.[4,9,10] Good nutrition is essential for maintaining good health, and a few principles are key in planning either a patient-selected diet or a portion-controlled diet. Nutritional quality of the diet, and obesity (a reflection of net energy intake) must be considered separately, because good nutrition can occur in either overweight or normal-weight people. Moreover, many overweight individuals have poor nutrition.

Dietary Protein

Dietary proteins provide amino acids for synthesis of body proteins.[4,9,10] The nine essential amino acids include histidine, isoleucine, leucine, lysine, methionine, phenylalanine, threonine, tryptophan, and valine. These must be obtained from dietary sources. The remaining amino acids can be synthesized in quantities sufficient to meet daily needs, except for arginine, which is required for adequate growth in many species. On a protein-free diet, which provides adequate carbohydrate and fat to meet energy needs, nitrogen excretion falls from

Table 4: Recommended Nutrient Intakes[5]

		Men	Women
Energy (19-50 years)	kcal/d	2,900	2,200
Protein (19-50 years)	g/kg	0.8	0.8
Calcium	mg	800	800
Magnesium	mg	350	280
Phosphorus	mg	800	800
Iron	mg	10	15
Zinc	mg	15	12
Iodine	μg	150	150
Selenium	μg	70	55
Vitamin A	(μgRE)	800	800
Vitamin D	μg	10	10
Vitamin E	(mgα-TE)	10	8
Vitamin K	μg	80	65
Thiamine	mg	1.5	1.1
Riboflavin	mg	1.7	1.3
Niacin	mg	19	15
Vitamin B_6	mg	2.0	1.6
Vitamin B_{12}	mg	2.0	2.0
Vitamin C	mg	60.0	60
Folate	μg	200	180

200 mg/kg/body weight/d (15 g nitrogen = 94 g protein) to a plateau of approximately 37 mg/kg/body weight/d (4 g/d of urinary nitrogen). Adding the small amounts lost in feces and from the skin yields a total of approximately 50 mg/kg lost per day, or about 20 g of protein for a 70-kg individual. This continued loss of nitrogen provides ammonium ion for excretion as a cation to replace Na^+ and K^+. The amino acids also provide carbon skeletons for gluconeogenesis.

Dietary proteins come from both animal and plant sources. The amino acid composition of animal proteins approximates those of human proteins more closely than do vegetable proteins. Thus, the quantity of protein in the diet from vegetable sources must be higher than when animal proteins are eaten. Moreover, vegetable proteins must be balanced across several vegetable groups to provide appropriate amounts of all essential amino acids. The Food and Nutrition Board of the National Research Council recommends an intake of 0.8 g/kg body weight a day of nitrogen to meet the requirements for more than 90% of the adult population, assuming that individuals obtain about two thirds of their protein from animal sources and one third from vegetable sources.[4] This translates to 45 g/d of protein for a normal 56-kg woman, and 56 g/d for a normal 70-kg man. When energy balance is negative, nitrogen requirements increase to maintain nitrogen balance. If 1 g/kg/d of nitrogen is required for an adequate diet, then individuals on a low-energy diet appear to need approximately 1.5 g/kg of protein per kilogram of desirable body weight, to provide maximum nitrogen sparing when other sources of nutrient energy are inadequate to provide energy balance.

A rough estimate of body weight can be obtained from the following rule of thumb:

Males: 106 lb + 6x [Ht(in) - 60] = weight (lb)
           48 kg + [Ht(cm) - 150] = weight (kg)
Females: 100 lb + 5 [Ht(in) - 60] = weight (lb)
           45 kg + [Ht(cm) - 150] = weight (kg)

For men - add 6 lb for each inch above 60 inches of height to a base weight of 106 lb.
For women - add 5 lb for each inch above 60 inches to obtain appropriate weight.

Dietary Fat

Dietary fats consist of triglycerides and sterols, including cholesterol. All cells, except red blood cells and the cells of the central nervous system, use fatty acids directly as a source of energy. During starvation, the brain adapts, using ketone bodies formed from fatty acids in the liver and transported into the brain across the blood-brain barrier. Dietary triglycerides provide both essential and nonessential fatty acids. Essential fatty acids include unsaturated fatty acids with two or three unsaturated double bonds. The most abundant essential fatty acids are linoleic acid and linolenic acid. They represent 1% to 2% of energy intake for adults, and 3% for growing infants and children. With higher-fat diets, linoleic acid may need to be increased. Omega-3 and omega-6 essential fatty acids, which have the first double bond beginning at 3 (omega-3) or 6 (omega-6) carbons from the methyl end, are oxidized by cyclooxygenase and lipoxygenase to produce prostaglandins and related products that modulate clotting factors and cell-membrane function. Some essential fatty acids should come as omega-3 fatty acids from either fish or vegetable dietary sources. Indeed, small amounts of these fatty acids from fish reduce the risk of sudden death from cardiac arrhythmia.

Nonessential fatty acids are generally the saturated or monounsaturated fatty acids. Saturated fatty acids tend to be solid at room temperature, and are associated with increasing risk of heart disease. Trans fatty acids also are nonessential fatty acids. Although they occur naturally to a small extent, most dietary trans fatty acids come from commercial hydrogenation of liquid triglycerides, such as corn oil, soybean oil, sunflower seed oil, etc, performed to make them solid at room temperature. However, the trans fatty acids produced by this process appear to have worse effects on the risk of heart disease than do the corresponding cis-saturated fatty acids.

Dietary Carbohydrates

Sugars. Sugars may be monosaccharide or disaccharide, and are largely found in fruits, syrups, honey, and as sucrose in many foods or on the table.

Starches. Starches are polysaccharides, and are the principal carbohydrates in cereals, flour, potatoes, rice, pasta, and other vegetables. The glycemic index has been used to subdivide the carbohydrates. The glycemic index is the rise in blood sugar after ingesting starchy carbohydrate, compared with that of a standard starch, usually potato. Foods with a low glycemic index (ie, absorbed more slowly) may be preferable as carbohydrate sources in overweight patients.

Fiber. Cellulose and cellulose derivatives in food provide fiber and roughage. Fiber is classified into two broad kinds: water soluble and water insoluble. The degree of solubility determines digestibility. Most cellulose-containing compounds are relatively indigestible unless partially broken down by heat or bacterial action. Dietary cellulose increases fecal bulk, and can be used as a laxative. Dietary fiber comes from seeds or skins of fruits, pulps of vegetables, and kernels of grains. Refining or processing of food often destroys or removes this fiber. Therefore, raw vegetables and fruits, in addition to whole-grain products, are preferable to processed foods as sources of fiber.

Carbohydrates should account for more than 50% of dietary energy. The rationale for this recommendation is based on the importance of glucose in several internal processes, and the value of a low-saturated-fat diet in reducing the risk of heart disease. Starvation lowers the activity of the sympathetic nervous system in experiments in animals and man. Dietary carbohydrate may stimulate insulin and help maintain the tone of the sympathetic nervous system. Dietary carbohydrate also modulates thyroxine deiodinase, the enzyme that converts thyroxine to triiodothyronine. In animals eating carbohydrate-free diets, the concentration of triiodothyronine drops. In the early phases of a low-energy diet, carbohydrates represent less than 50% of calories to maintain total protein intake. For maintaining weight loss, however, a low-fat, high-carbohydrate diet is recommended.

Vitamins and Minerals

Many vitamins and minerals are essential for human health. The Recommended Dietary Intake for many of these substances is shown in Table 4.[4,9,10] The recommended dietary intakes are based on the assumption that people eat 1,500 kcal/d or more. With diets of less than 1,200 kcal/d, providing all of these dietary components from natural foods alone is difficult. For this reason, patients on diets of 1,200 kcal/d or less need supplemental vitamins and minerals to provide daily replacements for these micronutrients.

The Nutrition Labels and the Food Pyramid

Nutrition Labels. All packaged foods now contain a useful food label containing important nutrition facts. One example of this format is shown in Figure 3 (low-fat milk). This food was selected for two reasons. First, it shows the nature of the nutrition label on all foods. Second, it showcases the use of the low-fat label, which means a reduction of more than 50% over the natural food. In reduced-fat foods, fat is decreased less than 50%. Skim milk, a third variety of milk, is fat free. The label has five parts. Part one describes the serving size, the number of servings in the container, the caloric value of a serving, and the number of calories from fat. The second part indicates the amount of total and saturated fat, cholesterol, sodium, total carbohydrate, dietary fiber and sugar, and protein in both absolute amounts per serving and as a percentage of daily diet containing 2,000 kcal. The third part lists five nutrients (vitamin A, calcium, vitamin D, vitamin C, iron). The fourth part shows the percentage of daily values in a diet containing 2,000 or 2,500 kcal. The final part of the label, at the bottom, lists ingredients in order of weight.

The Food Pyramid. To focus on the important dietary components, the U.S. government developed a Food Guide Pyramid in which the preferred components are at the bottom, providing the support base for food selection (Figure 4). Between 6 and 11 servings of bread, cereal, rice,

LOWFAT MILK

NUTRITION FACTS

Serving Size 8 fl oz (240 ml)
Servings Per Container 8

Amount per Serving

Calories 100   Calories from Fat 20

	%Daily Value*
Total Fat 2.5g	4%
Saturated Fat 1.5g	8%
Cholesterol 10mg	3%
Sodium 130mg	5%
Total Carbohydrate 12g	4%
Dietary Fiber 0g	0%
Sugars 11g	
Protein 8g	

Vitamin A 10g	•	Vitamin C 4%
Calcium 30g	•	Iron 0%
Vitamin D 25g		

*Percent Daily Values are based on a 2,000
calorie diet. Your daily values may be higher or
lower depending on your calorie needs:

	Calories	2,000	2,500
Total Fat	Less than	65g	80g
Sat Fat	Less than	20g	25g
Cholesterol	Less than	300mg	300mg
Sodium	Less than	2,400mg	2,400mg
Total Carbohydrate		300g	375g
Dietary Fiber		25g	30g

Ingredients: Lowfat milk, vitamin A
palmitate, vitamin D₃.

Figure 3: The nutrition label. This shows the low-fat milk label, but is typical of all labels.

and pasta fulfill the recommendation from the bottom of the pyramid. Two to 4 servings from the fruit group and 3 to 5 of vegetables make up the second level. Two to 3 servings each are recommended from the milk, yogurt, and cheese group and from the meat, poultry, fish, dry beans, eggs, and nuts group. Fats, oils, and sweets are at the top and should be used sparingly, as should alcohol.[5]

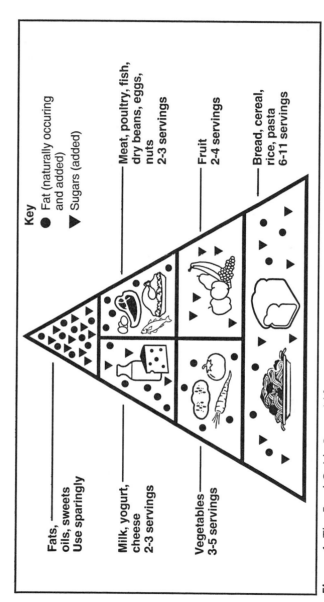

Key

● Fat (naturally occuring and added)

▶ Sugars (added)

Fats, oils, sweets
Use sparingly

Milk, yogurt, cheese
2-3 servings

Meat, poultry, fish, dry beans, eggs, nuts
2-3 servings

Vegetables
3-5 servings

Fruit
2-4 servings

Bread, cereal, rice, pasta
6-11 servings

Figure 4: The Food Guide Pyramid.[5]

Frequency of Eating

The role of altered patterns of eating in the development of obesity has been examined in both experimental and clinical studies. Classical experimental studies comparing animals allowed to eat multiple meals, to those fed identical meals by stomach tube, showed that the animals that received food twice daily by stomach tube had nearly twice as much body fat as did the animals allowed to eat at will. Clinical studies yielded similar results. Individuals who ate one or two meals a day tended to be more obese as estimated by skinfolds, as well as had higher cholesterol levels, than did individuals eating three or more meals a day.[2] Careful clinical studies have shown that cholesterol levels are significantly higher in those who eat a few large meals, compared with the same quantity of food eaten in many small meals. Thus, for a variety of reasons, we encourage patients to eat three or more meals daily. Breakfast is the most important of these. Individuals who eat breakfast are not as likely to be obese.

Questions About Diet

The following questions should be asked about any diet the clinician or patient wants to use:

- Does the diet have adequate protein? This means not less than 75 g/d for a low-energy diet.
- Does the diet reduce the intake of saturated fat and cholesterol?
- Does the diet provide adequate amounts of carbohydrates and starches—breads, cereals, pasta, and whole-grain products?
- Does the diet emphasize fruits and vegetables?
- Does the diet replace sugar with carbohydrate sources containing increased micronutrients?
- Does the diet recommend reducing sugar and alcohol intake?

Diets at Various Energy Levels

This section divides diets into three broad groups based on energy level (Table 1). The first group is diets with less than 200 kcal/d; second are the very-low-energy diets with calorie levels between 200 kcal/d and 800 kcal/d; and the third group is the low-energy diets with energy levels above 800 kcal/d, to any level 500 kcal below the patient's estimated energy needs.

Diets of Less Than 200 Kcal/d

Diets with less than 200 kcal/d can be viewed as starvation diets. The 200 kcal/d level is equivalent to 50 g/d of protein or carbohydrate or 22 g/d of fat. Studies in the early 20th century showed that humans can survive without food for more than 30 days. Starvation diets as a treatment for obesity were not popular, however, until the late 1950s. The enthusiasm for therapeutic starvation gradually waned for two reasons. First, these diets had many difficulties when used on an outpatient basis and, when patients had to be hospitalized, the high costs were a deterrent. Second, weight maintenance after the period of starvation was no better than other approaches, and body weight was regained as expected when any therapeutic regimen for obesity was stopped.

Therapeutic starvation produces rapid weight loss. Patients weighing 150 kg initially lose more than 1 kg/d, but this rate gradually slows to 0.5 kg/d after 3 to 4 weeks of starvation. Significant loss of sodium and potassium occurs during starvation, and has been associated with hypotension and syncope. Loss of protein with starvation also is significant. Urinary nitrogen excretion falls to less than 5 g/d from 15 g/d on a normal-protein diet of 94 g. A normal body uses approximately 150 g/d of glucose. After adaptation to starvation, this falls to 75 g/d. One third of this comes from glycerol released during lipolysis. At the beginning of starvation, protein provides the main source of carbon for gluconeogenesis. The conservation of glucose occurs by several mechanisms. First, the brain, which normally uses almost entirely glucose, adapts to consume ketone bodies by enhancing the blood-brain transport of ketones during starvation. Second, the increased concentration of fatty acids during starvation, along with lower concentrations of insulin, enhance fatty acid use as a substrate for conversion to ketones in the liver and for oxidation by peripheral tissues. Continuing nitrogen excretion may reflect a decrease in the availability of branch chain α-keto acids. Administration of keto acid derivatives to fasting subjects lowers urinary excretion of urea by providing substrate for transamination.

Several complications have been associated with prolonged fasting. Hypotension is common, and fainting can occur. Uric acid kidney stones have been reported. Thiamine deficiency has produced Wernicke-Korsakoff syndrome, and several deaths have been reported. Fasting, like other treatments that are not continued, has a poor long-term success rate.

Very-Low-Energy Diets, 200-800 Kcal/d

Very-low-energy diets are those with energy intake between 200 and 800 kcal/d.[11] The first reports on very-low-energy diets were published in the late 1920s. These diets, containing 1 g/kg of protein a day, almost completely prevent loss of body protein when they contain 400 kcal/d of energy. This observation was widely published in the 1930s, but failed to achieve continuing acceptance among the medical community.

Several different very-low-energy diets were introduced in the 1970s. They fell into two broad groups. The first group used foods, whereas the second used powdered or liquid protein diets. The early studies preceded a catastrophe after the publication of the *Last Chance Diet*. This book recommended a liquid protein supplement based on collagen obtained from the hydrolysis of gelatin, supplemented only with small amounts of essential amino acids. In 1978, the Centers for Disease Center (CDC) reported 17 deaths related to this diet.[12] The disaster with collagen-based liquid protein diets did not prevent the further use of these diets, but did raise cautions. First, prolonged use of any very-low-energy diet with less than 800 kcal/d can be hazardous. Second, use for more than 2 months or with a weight loss of more than 18 kg needs professional supervision. Third, the addition of carbohydrate and small amounts of essential fats appears highly desirable, if not essential.

Nitrogen loss with very-low-energy diets is affected by a number of factors:

- The length of time the diet is used. Nitrogen loss decreases over time on any diet that lowers protein intake. If the subject has previously been on a protein-restricted diet, the time required to reach nitrogen equilibrium on a given diet is reduced.
- Nitrogen loss is greater when the diet has less energy.
- The ratio of nitrogen loss to weight loss is inversely related to the quantity of body fat. That is, fatter individuals lose less nitrogen on a given dietary program of energy restriction.
- Most individuals achieve nitrogen equilibrium on a very-low-energy diet in 4 to 6 weeks. However, some individuals do not achieve nitrogen equilibrium, even over much longer periods of time.
- Even at very low energy intakes, a higher ratio of protein to total energy, within limits, reduces nitrogen loss.

The degree of sodium loss, in contrast to nitrogen loss, is influenced by the quantity of dietary carbohydrate. In addition to glycogen depletion, natriuresis is another reason for rapid weight loss on a low-carbohydrate diet. Also, a significant and early fall occurs in serum triglycerides. A significant decrease in serum cholesterol also is well documented in patients on very-low-energy diets. This reduction occurs primarily in low-density-lipoprotein cholesterol.

High-density-lipoprotein (HDL) cholesterol also may fall, even though it starts from a lower level. Very-low-energy diets have been effective in controlling type II (noninsulin-dependent) diabetes. A decline in serum triiodothyronine has been documented, and serum insulin levels also fall.

These descriptive studies allow us to reach at least three conclusions. First, on a very-low-energy diet, nitrogen loss gradually decreases, and many individuals achieve nitrogen equilibrium between 4 and 6 weeks. Second, the addition of carbohydrate to a very-low-energy diet reduces nitrogen loss over the levels achieved with the same amount of protein alone. Third, the protein should be high biologic quality. The presence of carbohydrates in a very-low-energy diet influences the pattern of electrolyte excretion and the metabolism of ketone bodies. One study, comparing the excretion of sodium in a very-low-energy diet with protein alone, showed that sodium lost was significantly reduced when glucose was part of the diet. Similarly, addition of carbohydrate reduces the degree of ketosis.[13]

The rate of weight loss on a very-low-energy diet is directly related to the degree of adherence to the diet. Weight loss has varied from 1.2 to 2.4 kg/week.[14] Weight loss plotted against the length of the study results in a straight line (Figure 5). This implies that effectiveness is high and that adherence is good. These rates are significantly higher than with the more conservative treatments. A 3-year follow-up of 192 patients who lost an average of 22 kg on a very-low-energy diet showed that mean weight loss 3 years later was only 3.3 kg. Of these 192 patients, 12% maintained 75% or more of their weight loss, and 57% maintained at least 5%. Exercise was the best predictor of success, and television viewing predicted weight regain.[15] In a 3-year follow-up, 58% of 74 patients who completed the 12-week program were more than 5% below starting weight and had improvements in comorbidities, thus meeting the Institute of Medicine criteria for 'success' (Chapter 5).[16]

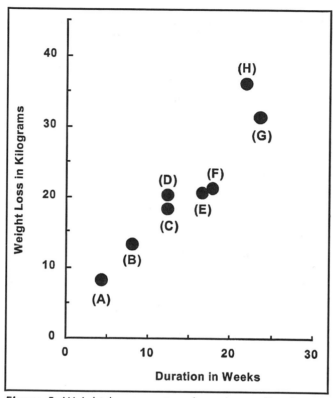

Figure 5: Weight loss on a very-low-energy diet. Degree of weight loss is related to length of treatment.[14]

Low-Energy Diets With Energy
Above 800 Kcal/d But Below Maintenance

Banting wrote the first popular diet book in 1863.[1] This classic pamphlet, which described how he lost weight and maintained the loss for an extended period of time, was the first of many 'How To' diet books. Low-energy diets come in all sizes and shapes. Some restrict one food or another, some have a balanced reduction in all foods but are low in energy, some are unbalanced in nutrient intake, some require ingestion or elimination of specific foods, and some require specific patterns of eating foods together or separately.

Evaluating Diets

The following principles form the basis for reviewing and selecting from the new and old diets.

- Select an energy intake significantly below maintenance levels to provide a desired rate of weight loss. A diet with a 500 kcal/d reduction below estimated energy needs generally produces approximately a 0.5-kg (1.1-lb) weight loss a week. A deficit of 1,000 kcal/d is anticipated to double this weight loss to 1.0 kg/week (2.2 lb). Figure 6 estimates rates of expected weight loss based on degree of energy restriction relative to need. This rate may initially be more rapid because of loss of glycogen and water.[17]
- Select an adequate protein intake. This should be more than 75 g/d of high-quality protein for a low-energy diet.
- Provide adequate carbohydrate intake because of its importance in maintaining activity of the sympathetic nervous system, maintaining normal levels of triiodothyronine, and minimizing ketosis, which can produce bone breakdown.
- Select a level of dietary fat that provides at least 3 g/d of linoleic acid or equivalent fatty acids.
- Reduce the intake of foods with high levels of saturated fats and trans fatty acids.
- Patients should eat no fewer than three meals and preferably five or more meals a day, including breakfast.
- Select from among a variety of foods, including those relatively high in fiber, with a preference for fresh fruits and vegetables, as well as cereals and whole-grain products.
- Women should consume at least 1,200 kcal/d; men, 1,500 kcal/d.
- Supplement the diet with a multivitamin and mineral capsule if the diet is below 1,200 kcal/d. Make sure calcium intake reaches the recommended daily allowance.
- Patients should avoid alcoholic beverages.

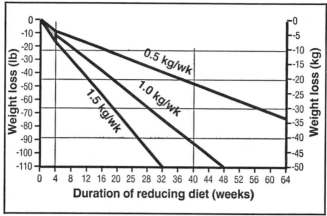

Figure 6: Range of rates of weight loss and duration of treatment.

- Patients should limit the use of fat spreads (butter or margarine), and use low-calorie items where available.
- Patients should avoid sugar-containing beverages.

These principles can be applied to a food diet based on foods purchased at a store, and to a portion-controlled food program using prepackaged or premeasured foods. The advantage of the latter approach is that natural foods are available and the quantity of energy is precalculated. Portion-controlled foods involve no guesswork. An alternative to a portion-controlled food program is one with a mixture of formula-based food and portion-controlled foods, such as canned or powdered products and many frozen foods. All food items must carry nutrition labels (see above), and these can be used to advantage in planning and following any diet.

Low-Energy Portion-Controlled Diets

Two broad dietary approaches can be used with overweight patients. The first is a calorie-reduced or balanced-deficit diet in which the patient focuses on counting calories; the second is a low-fat diet. Referring patients who prefer to focus on calories to a dietitian may be wise. Our clinic uses a

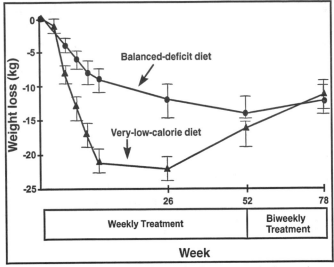

Figure 7: Comparison of weight loss on a balanced energy-deficit diet and a very-low-energy diet.[19]

portion-controlled approach to calories. Patients are encouraged to use a formula diet or diet drink at breakfast and lunch, and to use a portion-controlled frozen dinner at night. This helps keep calories under control. Individuals who wish to rigorously apply this dietary information can use a small scale and measuring cup to great advantage. This can be very useful and rewarding for some individuals who like to count calories, but the patient must have the long-term motivation to adhere to the plan. A menu-planning system is outlined in Appendix C, Guide to Better Nutrition.

Low-Fat Diets

The second approach is to reduce fat by counting fat grams. A fat intake of 20 to 30 g/d, if followed, increases carbohydrate intake. If this intake is from fruits, vegetables, whole grains, and cereals, fiber and dietary bulk increase. Food labels make it easy to count fat grams, and this is useful for many patients.

222

In a group of 238 patients who selected their own treatment, those choosing liquid-formula diets lost more weight in the first 24 weeks, but by 40 weeks they had no different weight loss than those using an individualized food diet, with or without medications.[18] In a 78-week (18-month) trial, Wadden et al compared a very-low-energy diet and a balanced-deficit diet (Figure 7). Treatment was weekly for the first 52 weeks and then biweekly for an additional 26 weeks. Weight loss initially was greater with the very-low-energy diet, but after 26 weeks this group began to regain weight and, by 52 weeks, weight loss no longer was different.[19] These data argue for balanced-deficit diets rather than very-low-energy diets.

References

1. Bray GA: Commentary on Banting letter. *Obes Res* 1993;1:148-152.

2. Bray GA: The obese patient. In: *Major Problems in Internal Medicine*, Vol. 9. Philadelphia, WB Saunders, 1976, pp 1-450.

3. Foreyt JP, Goodrick K: The ultimate triumph of obesity. *Lancet* 1995;346:134-135.

4. *National Research Council Recommended Dietary Allowances*, 10th ed. Washington, DC, National Academy Press, 1989.

5. U.S. Department of Agriculture: *Nutrition and Your Health: Dietary Guidelines for Americans*, 4th ed. 1995, Home and Garden Bulletin No. 232.

6. Rynearson EH, Gastineau CF: *Obesity*. Springfield, Charles C. Thomas, 1949.

7. FAO/WHO/UNU: *Energy and Protein Requirements*. Technical Report Series. Geneva, 1985, p 724.

8. Toubro S, Astrup A: Randomised comparison of diets for maintaining obese subjects' weight after major weight loss: ad lib, low fat, high carbohydrate diet v fixed energy intake. *BMJ* 1997;314:29-34.

9. National Research Council: *Diet and Health Implications for Reducing Chronic Disease Risk*. Washington, DC, National Academy Press, 1989.

10. Food and Nutrition Board, Institute of Medicine: *Dietary Reference Intakes for Thiamin, Riboflavin, Niacin, Vitamin B$_6$, Folate, Vitamin B$_{12}$, Pantothenic Acid, Biotin and Choline.* A report of the standing committee on the scientific evaluation of dietary reference intakes and its panel on folate, other B vitamins, and choline and subcommittee on upper reference levels of nutrition. National Academy Press, Washington, DC, 1998.

11. National Task Force on the Prevention and Treatment of Obesity, National Institutes of Health: Very low-calorie diets. *JAMA* 1993;270:967-974.

12. Sours HE, Frattali VP, Brand CD, et al: Sudden death associated with very low calorie weight reduction regimens. *Am J Clin Nutr* 1981;34:453-461.

13. Fisler JS, Drenick EJ: Starvation and semistarvation diets in the management of obesity. *Annu Rev Nutr* 1987;7:465-484.

14. Wadden TA, Stunkard AJ, Brownell KD: Very low calorie diets: their efficacy, safety, and future. *Ann Intern Med* 1983;99:675-684.

15. Grodstein F, Levine R, Troy L, et al: Three-year follow-up of participants in a commercial weight loss program. Can you keep it off? *Arch Intern Med* 1996;156:1302-1306.

16. Ellrott T, Olschewki P, Jalkanen L, et al: Comparable evaluation of obesity treatment using the new Institute of Medicine criteria of success: three-year follow-up of the German Optifast Program. *Obes Res* 1997;5:51S.

17. Garrow JS: *Obesity and Related Diseases.* New York, Churchill Livingstone, 1988.

18. Nonas CA, Foo ST, Pi-Sunyer FX: Comparison of different weight loss treatments over 40 weeks. *Obes Res* 1997;5:29S.

19. Wadden TA, Foster GD, Letizia KA: One-year behavioral treatment of obesity: comparison of moderate and severe caloric restriction and the effects of weight maintenance therapy. *J Consult Clin Psychol* 1994;62:165-171.

Chapter 8

Physical Activity and Exercise in Treatment of Overweight

"But wait a bit," the Oysters cried,
"Before we have our chat;
For some of us are out of breath,
And all of us are fat!"

— Lewis Carroll
The Walrus and the Carpenter

E xercise or physical activity is any rhythmic activity that elevates heart rate above resting levels and involves a large muscle group or the coordinated use of several large muscle groups.[1] Physical activity or energy expenditure is one component of energy balance, which underlies the pathogenesis of obesity and the overall principles for its treatment. Figure 1 shows the relationship of physical activity to the energy balance equation.

The various components of energy expenditure are shown in Figure 2. Approximately 60% of total daily energy expenditure is involved in basic, nonmobile activities, such as heat production for maintenance of body temperature, for maintenance of ionic gradients across cells, for beating of the heart, and for other chemical activities within the body. Only approximately one third of total daily energy expenditure is under conscious control and labeled as physical activity. The third component, rep-

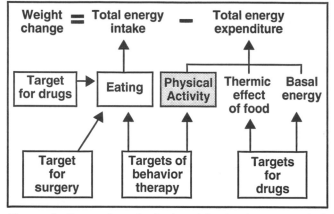

Figure 1: Target for physical activity in the energy balance equation.

resenting about 10% of total daily energy expenditure, is the thermic effect of food, which is related to both the composition and the amount of food eaten.

Measurement of Physical Activity

Measurement of physical activity, like measurement of food intake, is difficult.[2] Use of doubly labeled water, which estimates carbon dioxide production from the differential rate of deuterium and oxygen-18 loss from the body, provides the most effective quantitative estimate of total energy expenditure over 7 to 14 days (Chapter 2). With an independent measurement of resting metabolic rate and an assumption that the thermic effect of food represents 10% of total energy intake, an integrated estimate of overall activity over 10 to 14 days is possible. Unfortunately, this technique is only available for research purposes.

Alternative approaches to measuring physical activity have been developed based largely on questionnaires, using either the metabolic equivalent units approach

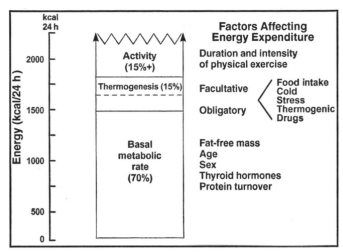

Figure 2: Components of energy expenditure.

(METS), or the physical activity (PAL) system. Accelerometers and pedometers are designed to measure movement. Heart rate measurements also have been used. Above the basal level, heart rate correlates well with energy expenditure characteristic for an individual.

Despite the limitations of these methods, estimates of activity clearly correlate inversely with health risks associated with obesity (Chapter 3). Also, unfortunately, Americans are becoming less active over time and with age. The Surgeon General's Report on Physical Activity found that the percentage of Americans participating in physical activity decreases as age increases[3] (Figure 3). Using the data from the National Health and Examination Survey (NHANES I), Williamson et al found that low levels of physical activity and recreation were strongly related to weight gain in both men and women.[4] For this 10-year study of weight change, subjects ages 25 to 74 were divided into two groups—those who gained more than 13 kg and those who gained less—and into

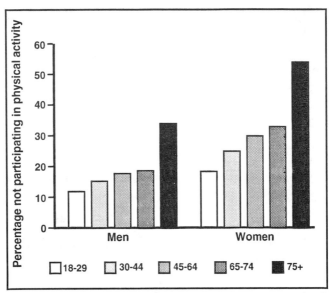

Figure 3: Percentage of adults not participating in physical activity by age group.[3]

three activity levels: low, medium, and high. Recreational activity was inversely related to body weight. Men and women in the low-activity category were 3.1 to 3.8 times more likely than the more active subjects to experience significant weight gain. Data from the Multiple Risk Factor Intervention Trial (MRFIT), as well as the Canadian Fitness Survey, also suggest that individuals who participate in vigorous physical activity have lower levels of body weight gain, skinfold thickness, and less abdominal fat as assessed by waist/hip ratio (WHR). In addition, a low baseline level of energy expenditure predicted weight gain in the Pima Indians.[5]

Benefits of Exercise

Exercise and physical activity have several benefits for overweight individuals.[6] The first is the well-known

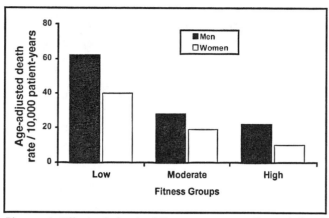

Figure 4: Effect of physical fitness on age-adjusted death rates (adapted from Blair).

reduction in cardiovascular risk that has been clearly demonstrated as a consequence of the physical fitness associated with exercise. Both Paffenbarger et al[7] and Blair et al[8] demonstrated the benefits associated with modest degrees of physical activity, compared with sedentary individuals. The Harvard Alumni Study found a graded reduction in death rates as the level of physical activity increased from less than 500 kcal/week to more than 2,000 kcal/week.[7] In the MRFIT, a physical activity level of 224 kcal/d significantly lowered the risk of death from heart attack compared with men who expended only 74 kcal/d. In the Lipid Research Clinics Study, the men who were least 'fit' were 8.5 times more likely to die of cardiovascular disease than were the 'most fit' men. An inverse relationship between physical activity and mortality also was reported in the Aerobics Center Longitudinal Study[8] (Figure 4). In addition to its benefits on longevity, physical activity also can increase well-being, and is known to increase sympathetic nervous system activity.[2,9,10]

Table 1: Activities Most Frequently Reported by the General Public[11]

Activity	NHIS		NWCR	
	Percentage Reporting Activity			
	M	**F**	**M**	**F**
Walking	39.4%	48.3%	78.6%	76.1%
Running	12.8%	5.7%	20.4%	8.2%
Cycling	16.2%	14.6%	22.4%	20.2%
Aerobics	2.8%	11.1%	4.1%	20.9%
Stair climbing	9.9%	11.6%	3.1%	9.5%
Weight lifting	20.0%	8.8%	24.0%	19.5%

NHIS = National Health Interview Survey 1991
NWCR = National Weight Control Registry

The second value of exercise is in maintaining weight loss. Several studies show the importance of physical activity in individuals who maintain weight loss. Individuals who are more physically active are more likely to maintain weight loss. This is shown in Table 1, which compares percentage of the general public reporting various types of physical activity, with individuals in the National Weight Control Registry who maintained a weight loss of at least 13.6 kg for at least 1 year. Except for stair climbing, a higher percentage of the formerly obese were in each active category.[11] Higher levels of physical activity and fitness also predict positive mental health status, enhance self-esteem and general self-efficacy, and reduce stress.[12] One of the most instructive examples is the study of diet plus exercise in a short-term, 8-week study with an 18-month follow-up[13] (Figure 5). During the initial comparison of diet and diet plus exercise, weight losses were not significantly different in this group of policemen. However, during follow-up, the impact of exercise is immediately apparent. Individuals who maintained activity levels had minimal weight regain. Individuals who stopped exercising gained weight and, if they started to exercise again, their weight declined. Men who were initially physically active but who became inactive experienced a sharp increase in body weight.

Exercise as a Sole Treatment for Obesity

Zachwieja summarized the effect on weight loss of five exercise programs without diet (Table 2).[1] Weight losses generally were quite small, except in individuals in military training. In three other meta-analyses, weight losses averaged 0.1 kg/week.[14-16]

Exercise and Diet Combined in Treatment for Obesity

Exercise programs added to diets with moderate to severe caloric restriction show no consistent additional effect on weight loss.[6] Warwick and Garrow compared three women observed for 12 weeks on a metabolic ward while eating a constant calorie-reduced diet containing 800 kcal/d. They were unable to find any increase in weight loss when these subjects bicycled for 2 hours a day, compared with when they did no additional exercise. They similarly found no effects of physical training on nitrogen balance, and suggested that the failure to lose weight despite the greater energy deficit caused by exercise may have been attributable to glycogen deposition in trained muscles.

Effects on body composition also were observed by Pavlou et al, who randomized moderately obese policemen on a variety of reduced-calorie diets to exercise and nonexercise groups (Figure 5).[13] The officers who exercised for 20 to 45 minutes 3 times a week at 85% of their maximal heart rates showed no greater weight loss (11.8 kg vs 9.2 kg), but lost significantly more fat and less

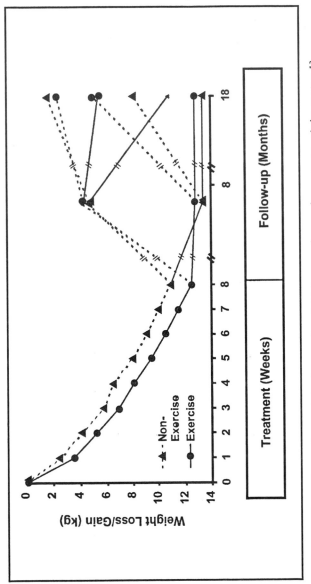

Figure 5: *Effect of exercise on initial rate of weight loss and on subsequent weight status.*[13]

Table 2: Effect of Exercise Without Diet on Body Weight Loss[1]

Meta-Analysis	Mode	Frequency	Duration	Weight loss
Epstein & Wing[14]	Walk/run	2x-5x/week	6-20 weeks	0.09 kg/week
Ballor & Keesey[15]	Walk/run/cycle	3x-4x/week	avg. 16.8 weeks	0.1 kg/week
Garrow & Summerbell[16]	Walk/run/cycle	3x-4x/week	8-52 weeks	0.1 kg/week
Original Investigations				
Hadjiolova et al[17]	Various physical activities & sports	Daily	45 days	0.6 kg/week
Lee et al[18]	Military training	5 days/week	5 months	1.8 kg/week

lean body mass than did the nonexercise group. However, other studies failed to demonstrate a sparing of lean body mass by exercise during caloric restriction. For example, Van Dale randomly assigned 6 of 12 obese females on a 12-week restricted-calorie diet of approximately 800 kcal/d to exercise for 1 hour, 4 days a week at 50% to 60% of their maximum aerobic capacity. Both groups lost 12 to 13 kg, but no differences occurred in loss of body weight, body fat, or lean body mass.[19] However, some strongly suggest that exercise may reduce the loss of lean body mass during dieting, though research is contradictory. Factors such as sex, age, quality and type of diet, and frequency and intensity of exercise, may explain some of the discrepancies.

Table 3: Body Composition Changes in Obese Adults After Diet, Exercise, or Diet Plus Exercise Intervention[21]

Variable	Diet (D)[a]	Exercise (E)[a]	Diet + Exercise (DE)[a]
Weight lost (kg)	10.7 ± 0.5 (269)	2.9 ± 0.4[c-f] (90)	11.0 ± 0.6 (134)
Percentage body fat decrease	6.0 ± 1.0 (46)	3.5 ± 0.5[c,e,f] (56)	7.3 ± 0.8 (43)
Weight loss maintained at 1 year[b]	6.6 ± 0.5 (91)	6.1 ± 2.1 (7)	8.6 ± 0.8 (54)

Data are means ± s.e.m.

[a]Number in parentheses represents the number of studies reporting data for that particular variable. This number may vary for the covariate analyses if a study did not report data for the covariate in question.

[b]Not enough studies included data for a covariate analysis using initial percentage body fat or initial BMI as the covariate.

[c]Significantly different from other programs when ANOVA was run without covariates.

[d]Significantly different from other programs when analysis was run with initial body weight as covariate.

[e]Significantly different from other programs when analysis was run with initial percentage body fat as a covariate.

[f]Significantly different from other programs when analysis was run with initial BMI as a covariate.

Maintenance of Weight Loss

Several studies with long-term follow-up suggest that including exercise in a weight-control program leads to improved long-term results.[2,6,12,21,22] One recent study assigned 128 women to one of four groups, which allowed for comparison of two different kinds of exercise over 48 weeks when they all received the same behavior program.[20]

Table 4: ACSM Guidelines for Medical Examination and Diagnostic Exercise Testing Before Beginning an Exercise Program[9]

	Apparently Healthy		Higher Risk[a]		
Medical examination and diagnostic exercise test recommended before:	Age ≤40 years (men) ≤50 years (women)	Age >40 years (men) >50 years (women)	No symptoms	Symptoms	With disease[b]
Moderate exercise[c]	No	No	No	Yes	Yes
Vigorous exercise[d]	No	Yes	Yes	Yes	Yes

[a] Individuals with 2 or more coronary risk factors or symptoms.
[b] Individuals with known cardiac, pulmonary, or metabolic disease.
[c] Exercise intensity well within the individual's capacity and that can be comfortably sustained for prolonged periods (eg, 60 minutes). Exercise should progress slowly and be generally noncompetitive.
[d] Exercise intense enough to represent a substantial challenge and that would ordinarily result in fatigue within 20 minutes.
Adapted from: American College of Sports Medicine, Preventive and Rehabilitative Exercise Committee: *Guidelines for Exercise Testing and Prescription*, 4th ed. Philadelphia, Lea & Febiger, 1991. Used with permission.

One group had diet only, a second had diet plus aerobic training, a third had diet plus strength training, and the final group had diet plus exercise modalities. By week 24, average weight loss was 16.5 kg (36.3 lb), and further weight loss continued over the next 24 weeks. The women who participated in the aerobic program had a smaller fall in resting energy expenditure, but no differences occurred

Table 5: Heart Rates (Beats/Minute) According to Age*[9]

Age (years)	55% of maximum[a]
20	110
25	107
30	104
35	102
40	99
45	96
50	93
55	91
60	88
65	85
70	82
75	80
80	77

* This formula is only an approximation of any individual's response, and does not apply when certain rate-altering medications are being taken, such as beta-blockers and some calcium antagonists.
[a] Minimum exercise heart rate for health benefit designated by ACSM.
[b] Minimum exercise heart rate for fitness designated by ACSM.
[c] Maximum exercise heart rate designated for ACSM.
[d] Maximum average heart rate adjusted for age (according to formula: maximum = 220 - age).

among groups in body composition or weight loss, nor were there differences in appetite or mood. Exercise thus added little to the overall dietary program.

A recent meta-analysis of diet, exercise, and the combination of diet and exercise leads to similar conclusions, but also allows for comparison of the effect of exercise alone. The review included 493 studies from a total of more

60% of maximum[b]	90% of maximum[c]	Maximum[d]
120	180	200
117	177	195
114	173	190
111	168	185
108	163	180
105	159	175
102	153	170
99	149	165
96	143	160
93	140	155
90	135	150
87	132	145
84	129	140

Adapted from: American College of Sports Medicine, Preventive and Rehabilitative Exercise Committee. *Guidelines for Exercise Testing and Prescription*, 4th ed. Philadelphia, Lea & Febiger, 1991. Used with permission.

than 700.[21] Only aerobic exercise was included. Most studies were short term, lasting 15 weeks, and included moderately overweight individuals with a body mass index (BMI) of 33.4 and an average weight of 92.7 kg. The subjects who participated in exercise alone lost 2.9 ± 0.4 kg, compared with 10.7 ± 0.5 kg for the diet-only group, and 11.0 kg ± 0.6 kg for the combination of diet and exercise. Table 3 compares the 1-year results of this meta-analysis. The diet and exercise group weighed 8.6 ± 0.8 kg less 1 year later and the diet-only group weighed 6.6 ± 0.5 kg less, indicating the value of an exercise program in helping maintain weight loss. Exercise consistently stands out as a significant factor in maintaining weight loss after any program.[22,23]

A Program for Physical Activity

Increasing physical activity is beneficial for all ages and all groups.[1,4,5] Determining patients' general level of activity is important. Patients should be encouraged to spend 20 to 30 minutes or more in activity at least 5 days a week. The organized activities in which they normally engage should be identified, and increased participation should be encouraged.

Before beginning any exercise program, make sure that older individuals and those with a family history of cardiovascular disease do not already have impaired coronary circulation. The criteria for assessment are shown in Table 4.[9] Concern about cardiovascular risk should be addressed with a treadmill test. The level of acceptable heart rate elevation in relation to age is shown in Table 5.[9] Any exercise program should be designed to fit into the health and physical condition of the patient or client.[9,10] Existing medical conditions, age, and preferences for types of exercise should all be included in the decisions. Patients who are going to do exercise other than walking should be advised of the possibility of musculoskeletal stresses, strains, and joint injury (and even walking may produce these problems). Should joint or muscle pain occur, exercise should be terminated or reduced. In addition, climate can be important in activity, and appropriate fluid intake is essential.

Physical activity should be increased to 20 to 30 minutes, 5 to 7 days a week. One goal is to increase energy expenditure by 700 to 1,000 calories a week, or slightly more than 100 to 130 calories a day.[9,10] The amount of

Table 6: Calories Burned Per Hour of Physical Activity

Activity	Calories Burned
Shopping	150
Dancing	250
House cleaning, scrubbing, vacuuming	227
Walking (4 mph)	312

Two thirds of body weight expressed in calories/mile walking or running is a way to express energy expenditure in relation to body size.

energy expended in exercising depends on the duration, frequency, and intensity of the exercise, and on initial weight. A few examples are shown in Tables 6 and 7. Walking 4 miles an hour burns 312 calories (Table 6). This effect is related to body weight, and is higher in heavier persons. A 55-kg (120-lb) individual expends slightly less than 2 calories a minute more than standing still. At 73 kg (160 lb), this number rises to 2.4 calories a minute above basal expenditure, and at 91 kg (200 lb), rises to 3 calories a minute more than basal rate (Table 7). Thus, a 30-minute walk at 3 miles an hour for someone weighing 91 kg (200 pounds) dissipates an extra 90 calories, compared with individuals weighing 55 kg (120 lb) who dissipate only 60 calories an hour, or one-third less than the heavier individual. Because the amount of energy expended is related to body weight, if food intake does not rise, increasing energy expenditure to 2,000 calories or more a week is beneficial if the individual can do it. The time required to expend the calories contained in several foods is shown in Table 7 in relation to three body weights.

Table 7: Minutes of Walking to Burn the Calories in Various Foods

	Calories in Food
Apple (1) (21" diameter)	75
Apple pie (1/6 of 9" pie)	410
Beer (12 oz)	170
Blueberries (cup) (fresh)	87
Beef steak (cubed, 4 oz)	300
Bologna (1 slice)	88
Biscuit (1) (2" diameter)	130
Bread (1 slice)	65
Broccoli (cup)	50
Cola (8 oz)	100
Cooked cereal (cup)	165
Cheese (1 oz) (Gouda) (caraway)	100
Chocolate cake (1 piece) 2" x 3" x 2" (no icing)	165
Egg (medium)	78
Flounder (4 oz) (raw)	78
Frankfurter	124
Hamburger & bun (1 bun) (3 oz, high-fat meat)	400
Milk (whole) (8 oz)	166
Orange (large, 3 3/8" diameter)	115
Potato (baked-1) (no skin) (2 1/2" diameter)	100
Salmon (canned) (31 oz)	200
Strawberries (cup)	54

Minutes to Burn Calories Walking
at 3 mph
Body Weight (lb) (kg)

120 lb (54.5 kg)	160 lb (73 kg)	200 lb (91 kg)
21	17	14
115	93	78
47	38	31
23	19	16
83	68	57
23	19	22
36	30	24
18	15	12
14	12	10
28	23	19
46	38	31
28	23	19
46	38	31
22	18	15
22	18	15
34	28	23
111	91	76
46	38	31
32	27	23
28	23	19
56	46	38
15	12	10

Table 8: Energy Expended in Walking

Body Weight		Energy Expended (kcal)	
Pounds	Kilograms	5,000 steps	10,000 steps
88	40	100	200
110	50	125	250
132	60	150	300
154	70	175	350
176	80	200	400
198	90	225	450
220	100	250	500

An alternative approach for walking is shown in Table 8. The number of steps walked each day and body weight can be used to identify caloric expenditure. At 5,000 steps a day, an 80-kg (176-lb) individual expends 200 calories. An inexpensive step counter on the belt or waistband yields daily feedback on activity level. Step counters are available in many sporting goods stores.

In addition to being medically safe, any program involving exercise should be enjoyable, convenient, realistic, and structured.[9,10] Incremental increases in physical activity are easier to achieve than major changes done all at once. Such things as standing rather than sitting while on the telephone, or walking up one or down two flights of stairs rather than taking the elevator, are good ways to get patients started. Decreasing time in sedentary activity is a better strategy to get children and possibly adults to become more physically active.

Finding appropriate places to exercise facilitates any exercise program. The YMCA and YWCA can be useful, as well as health clubs, but for most individuals, walking is the most appropriate form of exercise, and can be done almost anywhere. In hot or cold climates, walking in a shopping mall is both safe and provides climate control. By adding 1,000 kcal/week of exercise, up to 12 kg of extra weight can be lost over 1 year if it is not offset by extra food intake.

In addition to its effects on assisting in weight loss, exercise has several other important metabolic effects that are beneficial to overweight patients.[9,10] First, exercise improves the capacity of the body to handle glucose loads. In a 29-month study by Tremblay et al, glucose tolerance tests were performed at 15, 21, and 29 months for comparison with initial values.[23] By the end of the program, even though these women remained overweight, glucose tolerance tests had returned to normal, as did insulin excursion in response to glucose. Prolonged exercise programs decrease abdominal fat more than they mobilize lower-body fat.[24] Improvements in lipid metabolism also are noted with exercise. The reduction in insulin and improved insulin sensitivity decrease very-low-density lipoprotein, the predominant carrier of endogenous triglyceride. High-density lipoproteins increase, and are more evident in males, probably because of the higher initial levels in females. Therefore, physical exercise and activity are important components of weight loss, but are particularly important in maintaining improved metabolic control and long-term weight loss.

References

1.   Zachwieja JJ: Exercise as treatment for obesity. *Endocrinol Metab Clin North Am* 1996;25:965-988.

2.   Hill JO, Saris WH: Energy expenditure in physical activity. In: Bray GA, Bouchard C, James WP, eds. *Handbook of Obesity.* New York, Marcel Dekker, 1997, pp 457-474.

3.   U.S. Department of Health and Human Services: *Physical Activity and Health: A Report of the Surgeon General.* Atlanta, Centers for Disease Control and Prevention, National Center for Chronic Disease Prevention and Health Promotion, 1996.

4.   Williamson DF, Madans J, Anda RF, et al: Recreational physical activity and ten-year weight change in a US national cohort. *Int J Obes Relat Metab Disord* 1993;17:279-286.

5.   Ravussin E, Lillioja S, Knowler WC, et al: Reduced rate of energy expenditure as a risk factor for body-weight gain. *N Engl J Med* 1988;318:467-472.

6.   Ballor DL, Poehlman EP, Toth MJ: Exercise as a treatment for obesity. In: Bray GA, Bouchard C, James WP, eds. *Handbook of Obesity.* New York, Marcel Dekker, 1997, pp 891-910.

7.   Paffenbarger RS Jr, Hyde RT, Wing AL, et al: Physical activity, all-cause mortality, and longevity of college alumni. *N Engl J Med* 1986;314:605-613.

8.   Blair SN, Kohl HW 3d, Paffenbarger RS Jr, et al: Physical fitness and all-cause mortality. A prospective study of healthy men and women. *JAMA* 1989;262:2395-2401.

9.   U.S. Department of Health and Public Services: Physical activity. In: *Clinician's Handbook of Preventive Services: Put Prevention Into Family Practice.* 1994, pp 311-317.

10.   U.S. Preventive Services Task Force: Counseling to promote physical activity. In: *Guide to Clinical Preventive Services*, 2nd ed. Baltimore, MD, Williams and Wilkins, Chapter 55.

11.   Thompson HR, Bear SL, Seagle HM, et al: Exercise behaviors in reduced-obese subjects in the national weight control registry. *Obes Res* 1997;5:84S.

12.   Institute of Medicine (IOM): Thomas PR, ed. *Weighing the Options: Criteria for Evaluating Weight-Management Programs.* Washington, DC, National Academy Press, 1995.

13.   Pavlou KN, Krey S, Steffee WP: Exercise as an adjunct to weight loss and maintenance in moderately obese subjects. *Am J Clin Nutr* 1989;49:1115-1123.

14.   Epstein LH, Wing RR: Aerobic exercise and weight. *Addict Behav* 1980;5:371-388.

15.   Ballor DL, Keesey RE: A meta-analysis of the factors affecting exercise-induced changes in body mass, fat mass and fat-free mass in males and females. *Int J Obes* 1991;15:717-726.

16.   Garrow JS, Summerbell CD: Meta-analysis: effect of exercise, with or without dieting, on the body composition of overweight subjects. *Eur J Clin Nutr* 1995;49:1-10.

17. Hadjiolova I, Mintcheva L, Dunev S, et al: Physical working capacity in obese women after an exercise programme for body weight reduction. *Int J Obes* 1982;6:405-410.

18. Lee L, Kumar S, Leong LC: The impact of five-month basic military training on the body weight and body fat of 197 moderately to severely obese Singaporean males aged 17 to 19 years. *Int J Obes Relat Metab Disord* 1994;18:105-109.

19. Van Dale D, Saris WH, Schoffelen PF, et al: Does exercise give an additional effect in weight reduction regimens? *Int J Obes* 1987;11:367-375.

20. Wadden TA, Vogt RA, Andersen RE, et al: Exercise in the treatment of obesity: effects of four interventions on body composition, resting energy expenditure, appetite, and mood. *J Consult Clin Psychol* 1997;65:269-277.

21. Miller WC, Koceja DM, Hamilton EJ: A meta-analysis of the past 25 years of weight loss research using diet, exercise or diet plus exercise intervention. *Int J Obes Relat Metab Disord* 1997;21:941-947.

22. Kayman S, Bruvold W, Stern JS: Maintenance and relapse after weight loss in women: behavioral aspects. *Am J Clin Nutr* 1990;52:800-807.

23. Tremblay AJ, Despres JP, Maheux J, et al: Normalization of the metabolic profile in obese women by exercise and a low fat diet. *Med Sci Sports Exerc* 1991;23:1326-1331.

24. Despres JP, Pouliot MC, Moorjani S, et al: Loss of abdominal fat and metabolic response to exercise training in obese women. *Am J Physiol* 1991;261:E159-E167.

Chapter 9

Drug Treatment of Overweight

*"I saw a few die of hunger;
of eating—100,000."*

— Benjamin Franklin

"To treat or not to treat—that is the question."
— with apologies to Shakespeare

D rug treatment for obesity has been characterized by therapies that have yielded disappointment. Beginning in 1893, almost all drug treatments for obesity have generated undesirable outcomes that resulted in their termination. Table 1 is an historical presentation of drug treatments for obesity and the side effects they caused.

An additional serious negative impact on the use of drug treatment for obesity is the negative halo spread by the addictive properties of amphetamine. Amphetamine, or **a**lpha-**m**ethyl-β-**ph**enethyl**amine**, is an addictive β-phenethylamine that reduces food intake. The addictive potential of amphetamine probably is related to its effects on dopaminergic neurotransmission. Its anorectic effects, on the other hand, are probably attributable to its modulation of noradrenergic neurotransmission. Because this β-phenethylamine is addictive, other β-phenethylamine derivatives were presumed addictive. Whether actually addictive or not, they were guilty by association. This has led to restrictions on the entire class of drugs by the U.S. Drug Enforcement Agency (DEA).

Table 1: Disasters With Drug Treatments for Obesity

Date	Drug	Outcome
1893	Thyroid	Hyperthyroidism
1933	Dinitrophenol	Cataracts, neuropathy
1937	Amphetamine	Addiction
1967	Rainbow pills (digitalis, diuretics)	Death
1971	Aminorex	Pulmonary hypertension
1997	Fenfluramine + phentermine Dexfenfluramine + phentermine	Valvular insufficiency

Drugs such as phentermine, diethylpropion, and fenfluramine (Pondimin®), and the antidepressant venlafaxine (Effexor®), are all β-phenethylamines. Phentermine and diethylpropion are sympathomimetic amines like amphetamine, but differ from amphetamine in having little or no effect on dopamine release at the synapse. Abuse of phentermine or diethylpropion is rare. Fenfluramine, on the other hand, has no effect on reuptake or release of either norepinephrine or dopamine in the brain, but increases serotonin release and partially inhibits serotonin reuptake. Thus, derivatives of β-phenethylamine have a wide range of pharmacologic effects. However, if examined uncritically, they could all be lumped with amphetamine and carry its negative halo. Thus, it is misleading to refer to appetite-suppressant β-phenethylamine drugs as 'amphetamine-like' except for amphetamine and methamphetamine, because of the negative connotations.

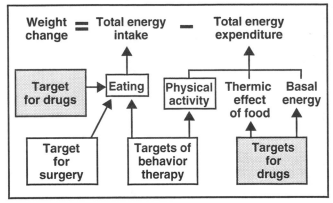

Figure 1: Targets for drug treatment using an energy-balance model.

A third issue in drug treatment of obesity is the perception that drugs are ineffective because patients regain weight when drugs are stopped. The truth is quite contrary. Overweight is a chronic disease with many causes (Chapter 4). Cure, however, is rare, and treatment should therefore aim at palliation. We do not expect to cure such diseases as hypertension or hypercholesterolemia with medications. Rather, we expect to palliate them. When the medications for any of these diseases are discontinued, we expect the disease to recur. This means that medications only work when used. This same argument supports medications used to treat overweight. Overweight is a chronic, incurable disease, and drugs only work when used.

Reports of valvular heart disease associated with fenfluramine, dexfenfluramine (Redux®), and phentermine posed the most recent problem for drug treatment of obesity. This is an example of the law of unintended consequences. The report of valvulopathy in up to 35% of patients treated with the combination of fenfluramine and phentermine was totally unexpected.

Table 2: Monoamine Mechanisms That Reduce Food Intake

Neurotransmitter System	Mechanism of Action	Examples
Noradrenergic	α_1-agonist	Phenylpropanolamine
	β_2-agonist	Clenbuterol
	Stimulate NE release	Phentermine
	Block NE uptake	Mazindol
Serotonergic	5-HT$_{1B}$ or 5-HT$_{2C}$ agonist	Quipazine
	Stimulate 5-HT release	Fenfluramine
	Block reuptake	Fluoxetine
Dopaminergic	D$_1$-agonist	Apomorphine
Histaminergic	H$_2$-antagonist	Cimetidine

The finding, however, will add caution to any future drugs marketed to treat obesity.

Targets for Drug Treatment of Obesity

Overweight results from an imbalance between energy intake and energy expenditure. This relationship was addressed in terms of a nutrient balance-feedback model in Chapter 2. The targets where drugs might be used in this model are shown in Figure 1. The feedback-nutrient balance model developed in Chapter 2 provides the framework for this approach to drug treatment. Drugs can reduce food intake, alter metabolism, and increase energy expenditure. This approach is used in addressing the available and potential drug treatments of obesity.

Table 3: Drugs That Reduce Food Intake

Drug Group	FDA Approval	Approved Duration of Treatment	DEA Schedule
Sympathomimetic Drugs Approved for Short-Term Use			
Norepinephrine Releasers			
Metham-phetamine	yes (warning box)	Few weeks	II
Amphetamine	yes (warning box)	Few weeks	II
Benzphetamine	yes	Few weeks	III
Phendimetrazine	yes	Few weeks	III
Diethylpropion	yes	Few weeks	IV
Norepinephrine Reuptake Inhibitors			
Phentermine	yes	Few weeks	IV

Trade Names	Dosage Form	Administration
Desoxyn®	5, 10, 15	10 or 15 mg in morning
Dexedrine®	5, 10, 15	5 mg 2 or 3 times daily
Didrex®	25-50	Initial dose: 25 mg once daily Maximum dose: 25-50 mg 3 times daily
Standard release: • Bontril® PDM • Plegine® • X-Trozine Slow release: • Bontril® • Prelu-2® • X-Trozine	35	35 mg before meals 3 times daily
Tenuate® Dospan®	25, 75	25 mg 3 times daily 75 mg once daily
Standard: • Adipex-P® • Fastin® • Obenix® • Oby-Cap® • Oby-Trim • Zantryl® Slow-release: • Ionamin®	37.5 30 37.5 30 30 30 15, 30	37.5 mg in morning 30 mg/d 2 h after breakfast 37.5 mg/d 9 a.m. 30 mg/d 2 h after breakfast 30 mg/d 2 h after breakfast 30 mg/d 2 h after breakfast 15 mg/d before breakfast (30 mg for less responsive patients)

(continued on next page)

Table 3: Drugs That Reduce Food Intake
(continued)

Drug Group	FDA Approval	Approved Duration of Treatment	DEA Schedule
Norepinephrine Reuptake Inhibitors (continued)			
Mazindol	yes	Few weeks	IV
Noradrenergic Agonist			
Phenylpropanol-amine	yes	——	——
Sympathomimetic Drug Approved for Long-Term Use			
Serotonin-Norepinephrine Reuptake Inhibitor			
Sibutramine	yes	——	IV

Reduction of Food Intake
Noradrenergic Receptors

A number of monoamines and neuropeptides are known to modulate food intake. Both noradrenergic receptors and serotonergic receptors have been the site for clinically useful drugs to decrease food intake[1-3] (Table 2). Activation of α_1- and β_2-adrenoceptors decrease food intake. Stimulation of α_2-adrenoceptors in experiments in animals, on the other hand, increases food intake. Direct agonists and drugs that release norepinephrine (NE) or block NE reuptake can activate one or more of these receptors, depending on where the NE is released. Phenylpropanolamine is an α_1-agonist that decreases food intake by acting on α_1-adrenergic receptors in the paraventricular

Trade Names	Dosage Form	Administration
Sanorex®	1, 2	Initial dose: 1 mg once a day Maximum dose: 1 mg 3 times a day with meals
Mazanor®	1	Initial dose: 1 mg once a day Maximum dose: 1 mg 3 times a day with meals
Dexatrim Accutrim	25, 75	25 mg 3 times daily
Meridia®	5, 10, 15	Initial dose: 10 mg/d Maximum dose: 20 mg/d

nucleus. The weight gain seen in patients treated for hypertension or prostatic hypertrophy with α_1-adrenergic antagonists indicates that α_1-adrenoceptors are clinically important in regulating body weight. Stimulation of β_2-adrenoceptors by NE or agonists such as terbutaline, clenbuterol, and salbutamol reduces food intake. The weight gain in patients treated with some β_2-adrenergic antagonists also indicates that this is a clinically important receptor for regulating body weight.

Serotonergic Receptors

The serotonin receptor system, which consists of seven families of receptors, also is involved in modulating food intake. Stimulation of receptors in the $5HT_1$ and $5HT_2$ families have the main effects on feeding. Activation of the 5-

HT_{1A} receptor increases food intake, but this acute effect is rapidly downregulated and is not clinically significant in regulation of body weight. Activation of the $5\text{-}HT_{2C}$ and possibly $5\text{-}HT_{1B}$ receptor decreases food intake. Direct agonists (quipazine) or drugs that block serotonin reuptake reduce food intake by acting on these receptors, or by providing the serotonin that modulates these receptors.

Altered Metabolism

Excess fat is the visible sign of obesity. Metabolic strategies have been directed at preabsorptive and postabsorptive mechanisms. Preabsorptive mechanisms that influence digestion and absorption of macronutrients were used to develop orlistat (Xenical®), which inhibits intestinal digestion of fat and lowers body weight.

The second strategy is to affect intermediary metabolism. Possible strategies include enhancing lipolysis, inhibiting lipogenesis, and affecting fat distribution between subcutaneous and visceral sites.

Increased Energy Expenditure

Increased energy expenditure through exercise is ideal for treating obesity. Drugs that have the same physiologic consequences as exercise would provide useful ways of treating obesity.

Drugs That Reduce Food Intake

Table 3 summarizes the effects of a number of drugs used to treat obesity. They are addressed in more detail below.

Sympathomimetic Drugs Approved by the FDA for Short-Term and Long-Term Treatment of Obesity
Pharmacology

The sympathomimetic drugs are grouped together because they can increase blood pressure and, in part, act like NE. Drugs in this group work by a variety of mecha-

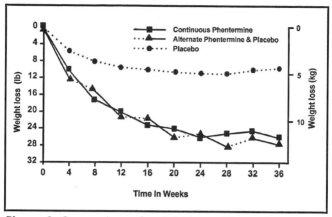

Figure 2: Comparison of weight loss with continuous and intermittent therapy with phentermine.[6]

nisms, including the release of NE from synaptic granules (benzphetamine, phendimetrazine, phentermine, and diethylpropion), blockade of NE reuptake (mazindol), blockade of reuptake of both NE and 5-HT (sibutramine [Meridia®]), or direct action on adrenoceptors (phenylpropanolamine).

All of these drugs are absorbed orally and quickly reach peak blood concentrations. The half-life in blood is short for all except sibutramine and its metabolites, which have a long half-life. Both metabolites of sibutramine are active, but this is not true of the other drugs in this group. Liver metabolism inactivates many of these drugs before excretion. Side effects include dry mouth, constipation, and insomnia. Food intake is suppressed either by delaying the onset of a meal or by producing early satiety. Sibutramine and mazindol have both been shown to increase thermogenesis.

Efficacy

The efficacy of an appetite-suppressing drug can be established by showing that, in double-blind, randomized clinical trials, it produces a significantly greater weight loss than placebo,[2] and that the weight loss is more than 5% below baseline weight. Clinical trials of sympathomimetic drugs before 1975 were generally short term because researchers widely believed that short-term treatment would 'cure' obesity.[5] This was unfounded optimism, but because the trials were short and often were crossover, they provided little long-term data. This section focuses on longer-term trials lasting more than 24 weeks, and on trials with an adequate control group.

Phentermine and Diethylpropion. A 36-week trial comparing continuous administration of phentermine with intermittent phentermine and placebo is shown in Figure 2.[6] Both continuous and intermittent phentermine therapy produced more weight loss than did placebo. In the drug-free periods, weight loss in the intermittently treated patients slowed, only to become more rapid when the drug was reinitiated. A small trial with diethylpropion showed greater weight loss than with placebo. Phentermine and diethylpropion are schedule IV drugs, indicating a regulatory classification as having the potential for abuse, although this appears very low. Phentermine and diethylpropion are only approved for use for a few weeks, which is widely interpreted as up to 12 weeks. Weight loss with phentermine and diethylpropion persists for the duration of treatment, suggesting that tolerance does not develop to these drugs. If tolerance did develop, the drugs would be expected to lose their effectiveness or require increased amounts of drug for patients to maintain weight loss. This does not seem to occur.

Mazindol. No long-term, double-blind, placebo-controlled trials have been reported with mazindol. In a 1-year, open-label trial, weight loss was 9%, which is comparable to weight loss with other sympathomimetic drugs.

Sibutramine. In contrast to all of the other sympathomimetic drugs in Table 3, sibutramine (Meridia®) has been extensively evaluated in several multicenter trials

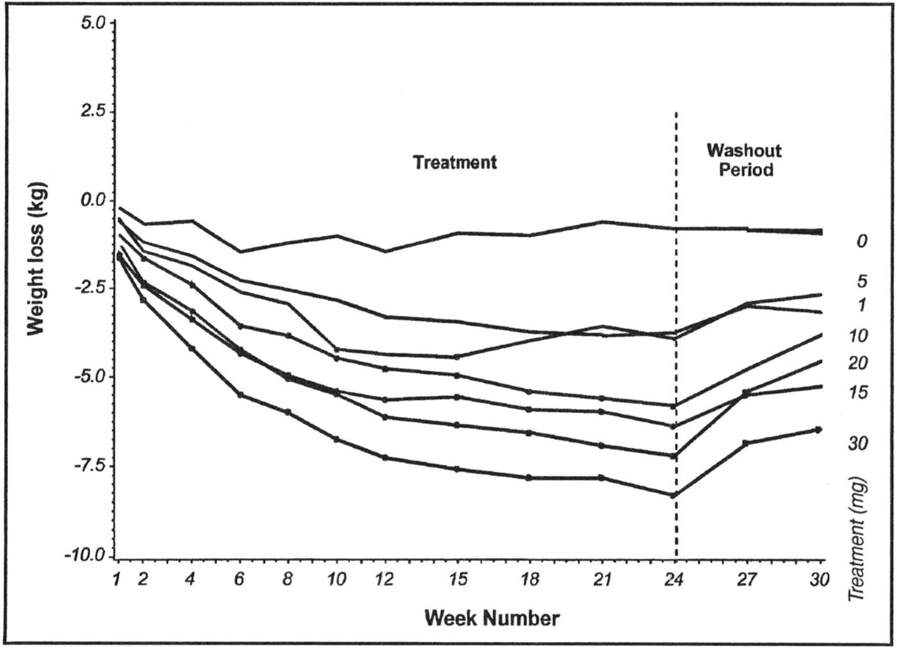

Figure 3: Dose-related weight loss with sibutramine. The regain in weight when the drug was discontinued indicates that it remained effective during treatment.[7]

257

lasting 6 to 12 months. In a clinical trial lasting 8 weeks, sibutramine produced dose-dependent weight loss with doses of 5 mg/d and 20 mg/d. Three clinical trials are included in the package insert. They were conducted in men and women ages 18 to 65 with a body mass index (BMI) between 27 kg/m² and 40 kg/m². In one trial involving 456 patients, 56% of those who stayed in the trial for 12 months lost at least 5% of their initial body weight, and 30% of the patients lost 10% on the 10-mg dose. In a dose-ranging study of 1,047 patients lasting 6 months, 67% achieved a 5% weight loss, and 35% lost 10% or more. The study found a dose-related reduction in body weight and body fat. Data from this trial on more than 1,000 patients are shown in Figure 3. The data show a clear dose-related response during treatment for 24 weeks and regain of weight when the drug was stopped, indicating that the drug remained effective. Nearly two thirds of the patients treated with sibutramine lost more than 5% of their body weight from baseline, and nearly one third lost more than 10%. The year-long trial showed that 10 mg and 15 mg produced significantly greater weight loss than did placebo, but that these doses were not different from each other. In a third trial, in patients who initially lost weight on a very-low-calorie diet before being randomized, sibutramine produced additional weight loss, whereas the placebo-treated patients began to regain. Lipids and uric acid were reduced across all trials in relation to weight loss. The medication is available in 5-, 10-, and 15-mg doses; 10 mg/d as a single daily dose is the recommended starting level, with titration up or down based on response. Doses above 20 mg/d are not recommended. Of the patients who lost 4 lb in the first 4 weeks of treatment, 60% achieved a weight loss of more than 5%, compared with less than 10% of those who did not lose 4 lb in 4 weeks. Combined data from the 11 studies on sibutramine show a weight-related reduction in triglyceride, total cholesterol, and LDL cholesterol, and a weight-loss-related rise in HDL cholesterol.

Safety

The side effect profiles for sympathomimetic drugs are similar. They produce insomnia, dry mouth, asthenia, and constipation. The safety of older sympathomimetic appetite-suppressant drugs has generated considerable controversy because dextroamphetamine is addictive. The sympathomimetic drugs phentermine, diethylpropion, and mazindol have very little abuse potential as assessed by the low rate of reinforcement when the drugs are available intravenously to test animals. Likewise, neither phenylpropanolamine nor fenfluramine showed any reinforcing effects, and no clinical data show any abuse potential for either drug. Sibutramine also has no abuse potential, but it is nonetheless a schedule IV drug.

Sympathomimetic drugs can affect blood pressure. Phenylpropanolamine is an α_1-agonist, and can increase blood pressure at doses of 75 mg or more. Phenylpropanolamine has been associated with stroke, and should not be used above 75 mg/d. Phenylpropanolamine has also been associated with cardiomyopathy. In the placebo-controlled studies with sibutramine, systolic and diastolic blood pressure increased by a mean of 1 to 3 mm Hg, and pulse increased by a mean of approximately 4 to 5 beats per minute. Caution should be used when combining sibutramine with other drugs that may increase blood pressure. Sibutramine should not be used in patients with a history of coronary artery disease, congestive heart failure, cardiac arrhythmia, or stroke. Two weeks should pass between termination of monoamine oxidase inhibitors (MAOIs) and beginning sibutramine. Sibutramine should not be used with MAOIs or selective serotonin reuptake inhibitors (SSRIs). Because sibutramine is metabolized by the cytochrome P-450 enzyme system (isozyme CYP3A4), it may interfere with metabolism of erythromycin and ketoconazole.

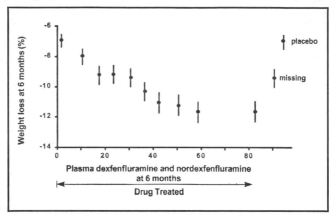

Figure 4: Compliance and weight loss with dexfenflura-mine.[8] (Abdalla and Pocock)

Sympathomimetic Drugs Not Approved by the FDA to Treat Obesity

Several other sympathomimetic agents either carry warning labels (amphetamine and methamphetamine) or have never been approved (fenproporex, chlobenzorex) by the FDA for treatment of obesity.

Nonsympathomimetic Drugs Not Approved by the FDA to Treat Obesity
Dexfenfluramine and Fenfluramine

Pharmacology. Fenfluramine (Pondimin®) and its dextroisomer, dexfenfluramine (Redux®), are serotonergic drugs that lack sympathomimetic activity but are no longer licensed to treat obesity because of their association with valvular heart disease. Dexfenfluramine, which contains all of the appetite-suppressing properties of fenfluramine, releases serotonin from nerve endings and blocks its reuptake. The d-norfenfluramine metabolite of dexfenfluramine acts directly on serotonin receptors, possibly the $5HT_{2C}$ type, to reduce food intake. These drugs are well absorbed orally, but have a long half-life in the plasma.

Efficacy. Fenfluramine was originally licensed in 1972 for short-term treatment of obesity. The International Dexfenfluramine (INDEX) study was a 12-month, double-blind, placebo-controlled, randomized clinical study of dexfenfluramine, and formed the cornerstone for FDA approval in April 1996.[8] Drug-treated patients lost significantly more weight than did placebo-treated patients, ie, 9% below baseline weight. Weight loss in the placebo-treated group also was noteworthy, a 7.5% decrease from baseline. When the patients were stratified by the amount of weight lost, 64% of the drug-treated patients lost more than 5% of initial weight, compared with 43% of the placebo-treated patients, and 40% of the dexfenfluramine-treated patients, compared with 21% of the placebo-treated patients, lost more than 10%.

The compliance data from the INDEX trial are very instructive. Dexfenfluramine was measured in the blood of placebo- and drug-treated patients after 6 months (Figure 4). Weight loss in the placebo-treated patients (right-hand point) was nearly 7.0%. In the drug-treated patients, weight loss was graded with increasing plasma concentration. Patients in the drug-treated group who had no detectable dexfenfluramine in their blood had a weight loss similar to the placebo-treated group, indicating that the drug does not work when not taken.

Safety. In addition to insomnia, dry mouth, asthenia, and loose stools, which are most prominent in the first 1 to 2 weeks of treatment and tend to subside, four serious problems have been associated with dexfenfluramine. These include pulmonary hypertension, neuroanatomic changes, the serotonin syndrome, and an atypical valvular heart disease that is addressed after the review of combination therapy below.

Primary pulmonary hypertension is a rare complication associated with appetite suppressant drugs.[9] Its spon-

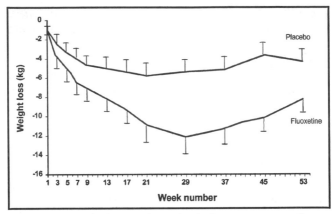

Figure 5: Weight loss and regain during treatment of over-weight patients with fluoxetine.[10]

taneous occurrence rate is 1 to 2 per million per year. Aminorex was the first β-phenethylamine associated with pulmonary hypertension (Table 1). It was initially marketed in Europe in 1967, and was withdrawn shortly afterward. Treatment with fenfluramine and other anorexigenics for more than 3 months has been reported to increase the relative risk of developing pulmonary hypertension by 20- to 40-fold based on data from a retrospective case-controlled study.[9] This is comparable to the risk of anaphylaxis from penicillin.

The neuroanatomic changes attributed to dexfenfluramine are a depletion of serotonin levels in the brain in experiments in animals. This was reported after treatment with high doses of dexfenfluramine given parenterally. The depletion is long-lived and blocked by serotonin reuptake inhibitors, which prevent dexfenfluramine from reaching serotonin storage vesicles. No functional impairments are reported to accompany the depletion of serotonin other than reduced food intake.

The serotonin syndrome arises when too much serotonin is released. It usually occurs when two or more sero-

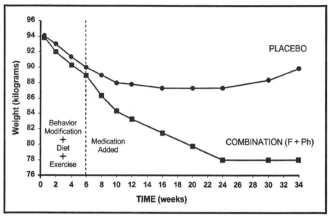

Figure 6: Effect of combination treatment with fenfluramine and phentermine. During the 6-week run-in period, both groups were treated with diet, exercise, and behavior modification. Treatment was randomized using minimization techniques to assure a close match at the start of the double-blind period. During the double-blind period, the placebo-treated patients lost almost no additional weight, whereas the drug-treated patients plateaued at a significantly lower weight.[11]

tonergic drugs are used concomitantly. It consists of altered mental status such as confusion, hallucinations, agitation, or mania. It also produces dysfunction of the autonomic nervous system with sweating, hyperthermia, shivering, and diarrhea, as well as neuromuscular abnormalities including clonus, hyperreflexia, rigidity, and tremor. Treatment consists of withdrawal of the medications and supportive therapy.

Fluoxetine and Sertraline

Pharmacology. Fluoxetine (Prozac®) and sertraline (Zoloft®) are highly specific inhibitors of serotonin reuptake into nerve terminals. They are readily absorbed and have a long half-life in the blood. Fluoxetine reduces food intake in experiments in animals.

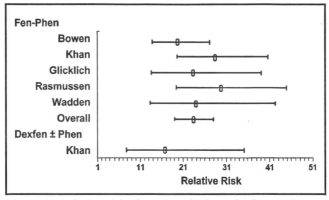

Figure 7: *Relative risk of aortic valvulopathy from echocardiogram-based prevalance surveys using CARDIA data as the reference (reprinted from FDA).*

Efficacy. Both fluoxetine and sertraline have been approved by the FDA for treatment of depression, but not for the treatment of obesity. In short-term clinical trials, fluoxetine produced a dose-related decrease in body weight. In longer trials, maximum weight loss occurred after 20 to 30 weeks of treatment. This was followed by a return of body weight toward baseline by 1 year (Figure 5).[10] In a trial with sertraline in patients who had lost weight on a very-low-calorie diet, the drug was no more effective than placebo in preventing weight gain.

Although fluoxetine has limited potential in long-term treatment of obesity, it may be valuable in treating binge-eating disorder (Chapter 4) or preventing weight gain in individuals who have stopped smoking.

Safety. Both fluoxetine and sertraline are widely used to treat depression, and have no significant safety concerns.

Bromocriptine

Bromocriptine (Parlodel®) is a synthetic ergot alkaloid that acts directly on dopamine receptors. It is most often used for treating pituitary tumors. Experimental studies show that modulating prolactin affects fat storage. Timed administration of bromocriptine is reported to reduce body fat and improve diabetes. Confirmation is awaited.

Cimetidine

Cimetidine (Tagamet®) is an H_2-antagonist that is widely used in the treatment of peptic ulcer disease. A small clinical trial showed that patients treated with 200 mg t.i.d. lost significantly more weight than did controls. More definitive data are awaited. The side effects of cimetidine are mild.

Combining Serotonergic and Noradrenergic Drugs
Efficacy

Drugs that act on either the noradrenergic or the serotonergic feeding system can reduce body weight. The possibility that combining serotonergic drugs with noradrenergic drugs might produce more weight loss or have fewer side effects with submaximal doses of one drug from each group formed the rationale for a 4-year, controlled trial of fenfluramine and phentermine.[11] The first double-blind, placebo-controlled portion of the trial is shown in Figure 6. During the baseline run-in, patients enrolled in an effective program of behavior therapy, diet, and exercise, and they lost weight. Patients randomized to drug treatment lost 15.9% from baseline, compared with the placebo-treated group, which lost only 4.9% from baseline. Some patients achieved long-term benefit by maintaining their weight at lower levels for up to 3.5 years, during which drug treatment was continued. This trial led to national enthusiasm for this drug combination. More than 18 million prescriptions were written in 1996 for this combination of drugs, and approximately 3 million to 4 million people were treated.

Safety

After this initial report, the use of the combination of phentermine and fenfluramine spread rapidly. In July

1997, 24 patients with atypical valvular heart disease were reported to the medical profession.[12] In the 3 patients in whom histopathology was available, the valvular changes were identical to the changes seen in carcinoid syndrome. By September 1997, the FDA had received reports on 291 patients, 92 of whom had valvular heart disease. Of these, 80% showed aortic regurgitation, and 23% showed mitral regurgitation. The relative risk of valvulopathy in 6 groups of patients examined echocardiographically, compared with the prevalence of echocardiographic changes in the CARDIA study, is shown in Figure 7. Based on the concerns raised by these data, both fenfluramine and dexfenfluramine were withdrawn from the market on September 15, 1997. An earlier report of cardiomyopathy developed during treatment with fenfluramine and mazindol went unnoticed, but may represent an early example of the same problem.

All symptomatic patients treated with fenfluramine or dexfenfluramine alone or in combination with phentermine are recommended to undergo echocardiogram. Because careful clinical examination fails to detect a murmur in more than half of patients with documented regurgitant lesions, an echocardiogram would be prudent for any patient who might need prophylactic antibiotics as recommended by the American Heart Association.

Peptides That Reduce Food Intake in Early Stages of Drug Development
Leptin

Leptin is a peptide produced exclusively in adipose tissue (Chapter 2). Absence of leptin produces massive obesity in mice (ob/ob) and in humans. Treatment with the peptide decreases food intake in the ob/ob mouse. The diabetes mouse (db/db) and the fatty rat, which have genetic defects in the leptin receptor, also are obese, but they do not respond to leptin. Leptin levels in blood correlate highly with body fat levels, yet obesity persists, suggesting leptin resistance. Clinical tri-

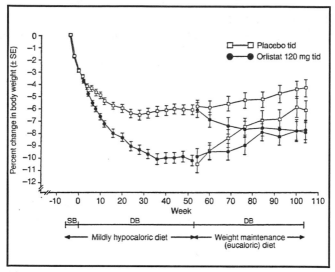

Figure 8: Effect of orlistat on weight loss during year one, and weight maintenance during year two.[13]

als with leptin are underway to see whether it can reduce food intake and body fat in overweight humans or diabetic humans.

Neuropeptide Y

Neuropeptide Y (NPY) is one of the most potent stimulators of food intake. It appears to act through Y-5 receptors. Antagonists to this receptor might block NPY, thus decreasing feeding. Early trials of one antagonist to the NPY receptor are underway, and more are expected soon.

Cholecystokinin

Cholecystokinin (CCK) reduces food intake in human beings and experimental animals. This effect does not require an intact hypothalamic feeding control system, but does appear to require an intact vagus nerve. Peptide analogs have been developed and tested, but clinical data have not yet been published. A second strategy to modify CCK activity is to reduce the degradation of CCK. This approach is likewise being evaluated.

Pancreatic Hormones

Glucagon. Pancreatic glucagon produces a dose-related decrease in food intake. A fragment of glucagon (amino acids 6-29), glucagon-like peptide-1 (GLP-1), reduces food intake when given either peripherally or into the brain.

Insulin. Circulating insulin levels directly correlate with body fat. Insulin level in the cerebrospinal fluid has been proposed as a feedback signal to reduce food intake. Infusion of insulin into the brain's ventricular system lowers body weight. A drug that reduces insulin secretion has been found to reduce body weight.

Amylin. Amylin is a pancreatic peptide released from the islet β-cell along with insulin. It also has been shown to decrease food intake and body weight in animals. Amylin lowers glucose and has been successfully used in Type I diabetes. Clinical trials on weight loss are awaited.

Drugs That Alter Metabolism
Drugs Awaiting FDA Approval
Orlistat

Pharmacology. Orlistat (Xenical®; formerly called tetrahydrolipstatin) is a potent selective inhibitor of pancreatic lipase that reduces intestinal digestion of fat. The drug has a dose-dependent effect on fecal fat loss, increasing it to about 30% on a diet with 30% of energy as fat. Orlistat has little effect in subjects on a low-fat diet, as might be anticipated from its mechanism.

Efficacy. Five long-term clinical trials with orlistat, lasting 1 to 2 years, have been presented in abstract form. The results of one published study are shown in Figure 8.[13] The trial had two parts. In the first year, patients received an hypocaloric diet 500 kcal/d below their requirements. During the second year, the diet was calculated to maintain weight. At the end of year 1, placebo-treated patients lost 6.5% of initial body weight, and drug-treated patients lost nearly 10%. Drug-treated

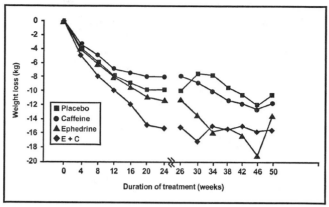

Figure 9: Effect of ephedrine and caffeine on weight loss and weight maintenance for one year.[14]

patients regained less weight in year 2 than did those receiving placebo. An analysis of quality of life in patients treated with orlistat showed improvements over the placebo group, despite concerns about gastrointestinal symptoms.

Safety. Orlistat is not significantly absorbed, and its side effects thus are related to the blockade of triglyceride digestion in the intestine. Fecal fat loss and related GI symptoms are common initially, but subside as patients learn to use the drug. Some patients also need supplementation with fat-soluble vitamins that can be lost in the stools. Absorption of other drugs does not seem to be significantly affected by orlistat.

Steroidal Drugs Not Approved by the FDA for Obesity
Androgens and Androgen Antagonists

Dehydroepiandrosterone. Dehydroepiandrosterone (DHEA) is a weak androgen that induces weight loss in several animal species. Clinical trials in humans have shown no effect.

Etiocholandione. Etiocholandione is a DHEA derivative that produced weight loss in one preliminary clinical trial. Additional trials are underway.

Testosterone. In men, testosterone and the anabolic steroid oxandrolone are reported to reduce visceral fat. A trial of an antiandrogen and nandrolone in women showed no effects on visceral fat.

Drugs That Increase Energy Expenditure
Drugs Approved by the FDA
for an Indication Other Than Obesity
Ephedrine/Caffeine

Pharmacology. Ephedrine is a sympathomimetic amine used to relax bronchial smooth muscle in patients with asthma. It also stimulates thermogenesis in humans. Caffeine is a xanthine that inhibits adenosine receptors and phosphodiesterase. In experiments in animals, the combination of ephedrine and caffeine reduced body weight, probably through stimulation of thermogenesis and reduction of food intake.

Efficacy. One long-term placebo-controlled clinical trial with ephedrine, caffeine, or the combination showed greater weight loss for the combination of ephedrine and caffeine than for either drug alone[14] (Figure 9). No other long-term data are available.

Safety. Although caffeine and ephedrine have a long record of clinical use separately, neither drug alone nor the combination is approved for treatment of obesity. Recent reports of problems associated with the use of ma huang, a natural source of ephedrine, raise concerns and it cannot be recommended until more data and FDA review are available.

β_3-Adrenergic Receptor Agonists
in Early Stages of Drug Development
The sympathetic nervous system is tonic in maintaining energy expenditure and blood pressure. Blockade of

the thermogenic part of this system reduces the thermic response to meals. NE, the neurotransmitter of the sympathetic nervous system, also may decrease food intake by acting on β_2- or β_3-adrenergic receptors (Chapter 2). Several synthetic β_3-agonists have been developed against the animal β_3-receptor, but clinical responses have been disappointing. After cloning of the human β_3-receptor, a new round of compounds is being synthesized that will be tried in obese humans.

Patient Selection for Drug Treatment

In Chapter 5, a risk-adjusted body mass index was developed to guide in the risk-benefit evaluation of overweight patients. Patients with BMI above 30 are potential candidates for drug therapy. Comorbidities such as dyslipidemia, hypertension, diabetes or impaired glucose tolerance, symptomatic osteoarthritis, or sleep apnea increase the rationale for treatment by shifting the BMI from 27-30 to an adjusted index above 30.

Sympathomimetic drugs can reduce body weight, but only sibutramine is approved for long-term use. This drug should not be used in patients with stroke, congestive heart failure, or myocardial infarction. The likely approval of orlistat will further expand the therapeutic armamentarium.

Weight loss of 10% to 15% can improve health risks. However, failure to lose weight or failure to improve comorbid conditions indicates either noncompliance with the drug or that the patient is not responding to the drug. Both require reevaluation of therapy and addition of other medications or other treatments. Patients treated with drugs should lose more than 2 kg (4 lb) in the first month, and achieve more than a 5% weight loss by 6 months. As long as weight loss is more than 5% and the patient's comorbidities have responded, the drug can be continued. The data with phentermine (Figure 2) suggest that intermittent use may be beneficial.

At least two groups of patients merit long-term drug therapy. The first are patients who are considered for surgical treatment of their obesity. Individuals with a BMI above 35 should first be treated with antiobesity drugs. If they respond with more than a 15% weight loss, drugs should be continued as long as they respond and comorbidities improve. The second group of patients who deserve vigorous treatment are individuals with sleep apnea. A modest weight loss often is sufficient to alleviate sleep apnea.

References

1. Bray GA: Pharmacological treatment of obesity. In: Bray GA, Bouchard C, James WP, eds. *Handbook of Obesity*. New York, Marcel Dekker, 1997, pp 953-975.

2. Bray GA, Atkinson RL, Inoue S: Pharmacologic treatment of obesity. *Obes Res* 1995;3:415S-632S.

3. Bray GA, Inoue S: Pharmacological treatment of obesity. *Am J Clin Nutr* 1992;55:151S-319S.

4. National Task Force on the Prevention and Treatment of Obesity: Long-term pharmacotherapy in the management of obesity. *JAMA* 1996;276:1907-1915.

5. Bray GA: Use and abuse of appetite-suppressant drugs in the treatment of obesity. *Ann Intern Med* 1993;119:707-713.

6. Munro JF, MacCuish AC, Wilson EM, et al: Comparison of continuous and intermittent anorectic therapy in obesity. *Br Med J* 1968;1:352-356.

7. Bray GA, Ryan DH, Gordon D, et al: A double-blind randomized placebo-controlled trial of sibutramine. *Obes Res* 1996;4:263-270.

8. Guy-Grand B, Apfelbaum M, Crepaldi G, et al: International trial of long-term dexfenfluramine in obesity. *Lancet* 1989;2:1142-1145.

9. Abenhaim L, Moride Y, Brenot F, et al: Appetite-suppressant drugs and the risk of primary pulmonary hypertension. International Primary Pulmonary Hypertension Study Group. *N Engl J Med* 1996;335:609-616.

10.   Darga LL, Carroll-Michals L, Botsford SJ, et al: Fluoxetine's effect on weight loss in obese subjects. *Am J Clin Nutr* 1991;54: 321-325.

11.   Weintraub M: Long-term weight control: the National Heart, Lung, and Blood Institute funded multimodal intervention study. *Clin Pharmacol Ther* 1992;51:581-585.

12.   Connolly HM, Crary JL, McGoon MD, et al: Valvular heart disease associated with fenfluramine-phentermine. *N Engl J Med* 1997;337:581-588.

13.   Sjostrom L, Rissanen A, Andersen T, et al: Randomised placebo-controlled trial of orlistat for weight loss and prevention of weight regain in obese patients. European Multicentre Orlistat Study Group. *Lancet* 1998;352:167-172.

14.   Astrup A, Breum L, Toubro S, et al: The effect and satiety of an ephedrine/caffeine compound compared to ephedrine, caffeine and placebo in obese subjects on an energy restricted diet. A double blind trial. *Int J Obes Relat Metab Disord* 1992;16:269-277.

Chapter 10

Surgical Treatment of Overweight

*"Our main business is not to see
what lies dimly at a distance
but to do what lies clearly at hand."*

— Thomas Carlyle

*"God heals and the
Doctor takes the fee."*

— Benjamin Franklin

Operating on overweight individuals carries extra risks associated with anesthesia, with intraoperative techniques, and with postoperative recovery. For these and other reasons, surgical intervention as primary treatment for obesity is relatively recent. The original operative procedures for treatment of obese patients were developed only 40 years ago[1] (Table 1).

The location where surgical treatment affects the energy balance equation is shown in Figure 1. Surgery affects only modulation of food intake by influencing the size of the gastric pouch or altering intestinal drainage. The rationale for the initial series of jejunocolic procedures was to temporarily reroute gastrointestinal contents to produce weight loss, after which the procedure would be reversed and the obesity 'cured.'[2] Metabolic problems, including loss of potassium and nitrogen, demanded early reversal. To the surgeons' disappointment, this temporary operation failed to cure obesity.

Table 1: Operations for Obesity in Humans[1]

1954	Jejunoileal small bowel bypass
1963	Jejunocolic bypass
1967	Gastric bypass
1971	Gastroplasty
1978	Gastric banding or wrapping
1978	Truncal vagotomy
1979	Biliopancreatic bypass
1981	Vertical banded gastroplasty
1981	Biliointestinal bypass
1982	Ileogastrostomy
1983	Intestinal interposition
1986	Esophageal banding
1986	Adjustable gastric banding
1990	Laparoscopic banding

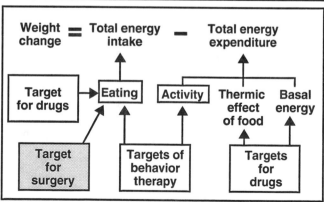

Figure 1: Target for surgical intervention in the energy balance diagram.

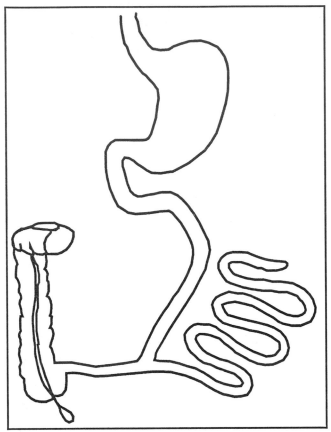

Figure 2: Common jejunoileal bypass.[3]

Recognizing that obesity is a chronic disease, therapeutic approach shifted to longer-lasting operative procedures. Surgeons coined the term *morbid obesity* to refer to the health risks in individuals weighing more than 150 kg (330 lb). The most common procedure in the 1970s was the jejunoileal bypass, using either an end-to-end or an end-to-side anastomosis[3] (Figure 2). The large

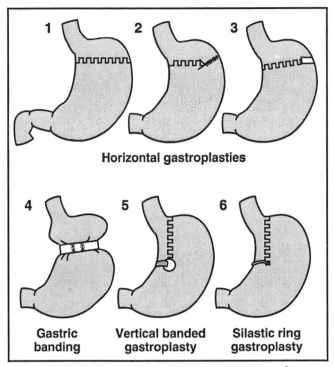

Figure 3: *Common gastric restriction operations.[5]*

undrained blind loop of small intestines led to a variety of metabolic changes, including liver failure, increased risk of uric acid kidney stones, and an immunologic syndrome primarily associated with arthritis. These problems led to discontinuation of this procedure. However, dramatic reports of improved functioning of these patients in both the social and economic spheres sustained enthusiasm for surgical treatment of obesity.[4]

Gastric Operations

Mason and Ito were the first to introduce operations to modify the stomach and its connection to the intestine.[6]

277

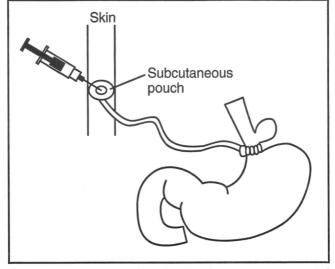

Figure 4: Laparoscopic band with subcutaneous reservoir.[1]

All of the procedures except the one developed by Scopinaro et al[7] are modifications of these gastric operations pioneered by Mason and his colleagues.

Gastric Restriction Operations

The first group of gastric operations are direct descendants of the gastroplasty procedure developed by Mason et al in 1971.[6] In this operation, sutures are placed across part of the stomach, leaving a connection between the upper and lower pouch. A variety of modifications with improvements were made possible by stapling machines and improved surgical materials. Figure 3 shows the common gastric restriction operations.[5] The most common procedure is the vertical banded gastroplasty (VBG). This is an elongation of the esophagus with a fixed termination midway along the lesser curvature of the stomach. To prevent this opening into the larger stomach from expand-

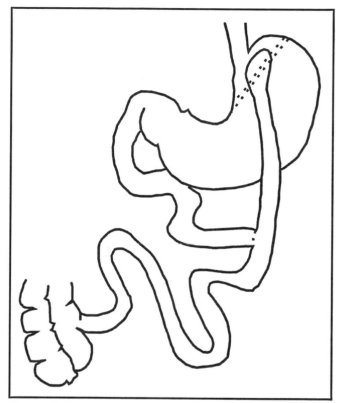

Figure 5: *Roux-en-Y gastric bypass.*[3]

ing, a number of banding materials have been used at the lower end of the extended esophageal path. In addition, some procedures use staple lines horizontally.

Gastric Banding

A second group of gastric restriction procedures wrap or band the stomach (Figure 3). A recently introduced gastric ring with an inflatable pouch placed subcutaneously can be introduced laparoscopically. With this procedure,

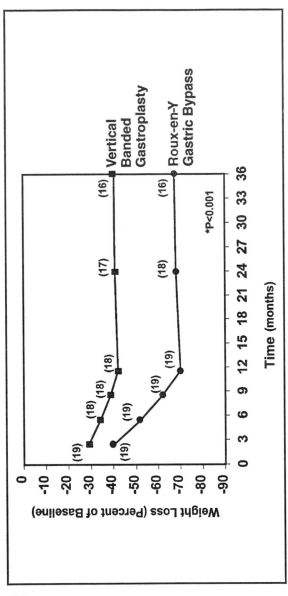

Figure 6: Comparison of weight loss in patients with a vertical banded gastric restriction operation (VBG) or a Roux-en-Y gastric bypass operation.[8]

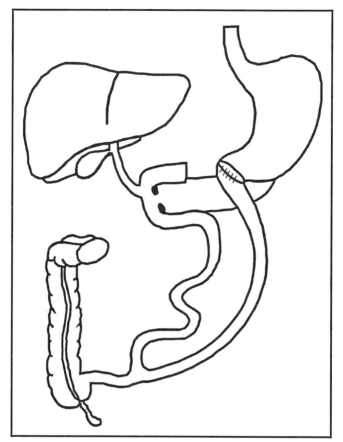

Figure 7: *Biliopancreatic bypass.*[3]

degree of gastric constriction can be increased or decreased by changing the volume of the subcutaneous reservoir that leads to the ring encircling the stomach (Figure 4).

Gastric Bypass

The principal gastric bypass procedure is the Roux-en-Y operation, shown in Figure 5.[1] Compared with VBG in randomized series, the Roux-en-Y gastric bypass produces more weight loss and, equally important, maintains that lower weight longer (Figure 6).[8] Food intake is reduced postoperatively, but the variability is greater in patients with VBG, accounting for the smaller weight loss. The possibility that food choices might influence success is supported by the finding that postoperatively, patients with VBG ate significantly more milk and ice cream than did those with the Roux-en-Y gastric bypass.[9]

Biliopancreatic Bypass

The biliopancreatic bypass is shown in Figure 7.[3] The stomach is transected and drained into the lower jejunum or ileum.[7] The duodenal contents are then emptied into the jejunum or ileum at a variable distance from the ileocecal valve. This operation produces some of the malabsorptive features that occur with the jejunoileal bypass, but avoids the complications of a blind loop. It is the most technically difficult procedure. The selection of the length in each limb can dramatically influence the amount of weight loss and degree of malabsorption.

Surgical Complications

A number of complications have been reported with these gastric operations (Table 2).[10] The operative mortality with all procedures is less than 1%. The technically demanding procedures, such as Roux-en-Y gastric bypass and biliopancreatic diversion, increase the risk of perioperative and postoperative problems such as anastomotic leak, sepsis, and pancreatic ulceration. Because of the diversion of intestinal contents, malnutrition occasionally occurs in patients with biliopancreatic diversion. Because the flow of gastric juice through the stomach and intestines remains intact, anemia is nonexistent with VBG, but is a rare problem in the Roux-en-Y gastric bypass. A peculiar variety of neuropathy that may be nutritional in origin can be associated with this. Anemia and malabsorption also occur with biliopancreatic diversion, depending on the length of the two segments of intestines in continuity. Surgical revision is common in all procedures. With gastroplasty, this usually occurs because of inadequate weight loss, which can run as high as 20%. In one series by the same surgical group, 6 of 30 patients with VBG had a revision, compared with 2 of 108 who had a Roux-en-Y gastric bypass.[9]

Benefits

Successful gastric surgery for obesity has a number of benefits. These include substantial and prolonged weight loss and improved quality of life (Table 3).[11,12] Employment record, satisfaction with reduced body size, and improved lifestyle are important for these individuals. This impact on the quality of life was demonstrated very clearly by Rand and Macgregor: "In spite of the proclivity for people to evaluate their own worst handicap as less disabling than other handicaps, (obese) patients said they would prefer to be normal weight with a major handicap (deaf, dyslexic, diabetic, legally blind, very bad acne, heart disease, one leg amputated) than to be morbidly obese. All patients said they would rather be normal weight than a morbidly obese multimillionaire."[12] Table 4 summarizes the impressive data on metabolic improvement from the ongoing Swedish Obesity Study.[13] In the first 2 years after surgery, risks of diabetes and impaired glucose tolerance were reduced. Benefits included reduction in blood pressure, improvement in lipids, and disappearance of sleep apnea.

Additional Operative Procedures
Lipectomy, Liposuction, and Plastic Surgery

Removal of excess skin and fat in individuals who maintain long-term weight loss can be beneficial, and was pioneered more than 50 years ago.[1] However, this procedure should be reserved for individuals with gastric surgery or

Table 2: Reported Complications of Common Surgical Procedures[10]

Complication	Vertical Banded Gastroplasty (%)
Weight loss (% excess body weight at 3 years)	40-63
Mortality (perioperative)	0-1.0
Leak/sepsis	0-1
Outlet stenosis	4-20
Peptic ulceration	1-8
Malnutrition	
Anemia	
Mineral/vitamin deficits:	
•iron	
•folate	
•B_{12}	17
Staple disruption	1.7-48
Surgical revision	41-45

Table 3: Benefits of Surgically Induced Long-Term Weight Loss

Surgical treatment improves:
- sleep apnea
- fertility
- urinary incontinence
- osteoarthritis
- pseudotumor cerebri
- quality of life
- employment opportunities

Roux-en-Y Gastric Bypass (%)	Biliopancreatic Diversion (%)
68-72	75
(55 @ 10 years)	(77 @ 9 years)
0-2.5	0.5-1.0
0-2.5	0-.3
3.5-22	3-5
2.2-11	2.8
	7
30-39	5-35
28-56	
1.8-14	
22-37	
1.6-8	—
1-10	1.7-20

some other procedure with long-term effectiveness. Otherwise, weight regain may lead to unsightly distortions in abdominal appearance, because fat is gained in one area and not others. Removal of fat by aspiration after injection of saline has been used as a plastic procedure to contour subcutaneous fat.[14] Many reports have been published on this as a plastic procedure for improving appearance, and it is beneficial. It is unacceptable as a quantitative method for removal of adipose tissue.

Vagotomy

In experiments in animals, vagotomy can reverse the obesity produced by hypothalamic obesity (Chapter 2).

Table 4: Improvement in Metabolic Risk Factors Over 2 Years After Weight Loss From Gastric Surgery[13]

Parameter	Men (n = 214)		
	Baseline	2 years	Δ
Age (years)	47.2 ± 5.7	—	—
Weight (kg)	129.7 ± 17	106.5 ± 19	-23.2
BMI (kg/m^2)	40.6 ± 4.7	33.3 ± 5.6	-7.3
Systolic blood pressure (mm Hg)	144 ± 18	137 ± 19	-7
Diastolic blood pressure (mm Hg)	91 ± 11	85 ± 10	-6
TG (mmol/L)	2.87 ± 2.4	1.96 ± 1.6	-0.91
Glu (mmol/L)	5.8 ± 2.3	4.9 ± 2.0	-0.9
Ins (mmol/L)	25.9 ± 14.8	13.7 ± 9.3	-12.2
Uric (μmol/L)	419 ± 82	358 ± 90	-61
Cholesterol (mmol/L)	6.1 ± 1.2	5.6 ± 1.2	-0.5
High-density lipoprotein cholesterol (mmol/L)	1.06 ± 0.23	1.18 ± 0.30	+0.12

With this experimental background, Kral evaluated the effect of truncal vagotomy in massively overweight subjects.[15] The results at 1 year were promising, but were largely overcome by weight regain 5 years after the operation. Adding vagotomy to VBG, however, increased weight loss by approximately 20%, suggesting that it may be useful to add to this procedure.

	Women (n = 241)	
Baseline	**2 years**	Δ
47.6 ± 6.0	—	—
113.8 ± 14	93.5 ± 17	-26.3
42.0 ± 4.0	34.5 ± 5.8	-7.5
144 ± 19	137 ± 19	-7
88 ± 11	83 ± 9.5	-5
2.08 ± 1.2	1.67 ± 1.0	-0.41
5.5 ± 2.1	4.7 ± 1.7	-0.8
20.7 ± 11.8	11.6 ± 7.7	-9.1
356 ± 80	295 ± 76	-61
5.9 ± 1.1	5.8 ± 1.1	-0.1
1.23 ± 0.29	1.35 ± 0.32	+0.12

Jaw Wiring

Dental splinting of upper and lower jaws is well known as a treatment for mandibular fracture. Several reports, mostly in the 1980s, evaluated the effects of dental splinting as a treatment for obesity.[1,3] In a long-term trial by Bjorvell and Rossner, jaw wiring was maintained for 6 months and compared with intensive behavior treatment.[16]

During the period of jaw wiring, patients lost more than 50% of the excess weight, compared with 40% of the excess weight for the behavior therapy group. However, after removal of the dental splints and introduction of behavior therapy, maintenance of weight loss by the two groups converged to about 30% of the excess weight (Chapter 6). In an effort to improve this outcome, Garrow and Gardiner introduced a waist cord, which he positioned in a group of individuals who had lost 31.8 kg during jaw wiring.[17] In a 4- to 14-month follow-up, they regained only 5.6 kilograms. Although jaw wiring, like all other treatments, is followed by rapid weight regain when ended, the possibility of continuing treatment in the form of an ever-present waist cord may add a novel dimension to this strategy.

Intragastric Balloons

Trials from two different types of intragastric balloons have been reported. Although the initial uncontrolled data were promising, subsequent controlled trials with balloons show that they are not effective in producing weight loss.[3]

References

1. Kral JG: Surgical treatment of obesity. In: Bray GA, Bouchard C, James WP, eds. *Handbook of Obesity*. New York, Marcel Dekker, 1997, pp 977-993.

2. Payne JH, DeWind LT, Commons RR: Metabolic observations in patients with jejunocolic shunts. *Am J Surg* 1963;106: 273-289.

3. Greenway FL: Surgery for obesity. *Endocrinol Metab Clin North Am* 1996;25:1005-1027.

4. Solow C, Silberfarb PM, Swift K: Psychological effects of intestinal bypass surgery for severe obesity. *N Engl J Med* 1974;290:300-304.

5. Grace DM: Gastric restriction procedures for treating severe obesity. *Am J Clin Nutr* 1992;55:556S-559S.

6. Mason EE, Ito C: Gastric bypass. *Ann Surg* 1969;170: 329-339.

7.   Scopinaro N, Gianetta E, Civalleri D, et al: Partial and total biliopancreatic bypass in the surgical treatment of obesity. *Int J Obes* 1981;5:421-429.

8.   Sugerman HJ, Kellum JM, Engle KM, et al: Gastric bypass for treating severe obesity. *Am J Clin Nutr* 1992;55:560S-566S.

9.   Brolin RL, Robertson LB, Kenler HA, et al: Weight loss and dietary intake after vertical banded gastroplasty and Roux-en-Y gastric bypass. *Ann Surg* 1994;220:782-790.

10.   American Obesity Association and Shape Up America!: Guidance for treatment of adult obesity, 1996.

11.   Proceedings of a National Institutes of Health Consensus Development Conference. March 25-27, 1991, Bethesda, MD. Gastrointestinal surgery for severe obesity. *Am J Clin Nutr* 1992;55:487S-619S.

12.   Rand CS, Macgregor AM: Successful weight loss following obesity surgery and the perceived liability of morbid obesity. *Int J Obes* 1991;15:577-579.

13.   Sjostrom CD, Lissner L, Sjostrom L: Relationships between changes in body composition and changes in cardiovascular risk factors: the SOS Intervention study. Swedish Obese Subjects. *Obes Res* 1997;5:519-530.

14.   Ersek RA, Zambrano J, Surak GS, et al: Suction-assisted lipectomy for correction of 202 figure faults in 101 patients: indications, limitations, and applications. *Plast Reconstr Surg* 1986;78:615-626.

15.   Kral JG: Vagotomy for treatment of severe obesity. *Lancet* 1978;1:307-308.

16.   Bjorvell H, Rossner S: Long term treatment of severe obesity: four year follow up of combined behavioural modification programme. *Br Med J (Clin Res Ed)* 1985;291:379-382.

17.   Garrow JS, Gardiner GT: Maintenance of weight loss in obese patients after jaw wiring. *Br Med J (Clin Res Ed)* 1981;282:858-860.

Appendix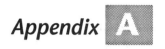

The Dieting Readiness Test

Answer the questions below to see how well your attitudes equip you for a weight loss program. For each question, circle the answer that best describes your attitude. As you complete each of the six sections, add the numbers of your answers and compare them with the scoring guide at the end of each section.

Section 1: Goals and Attitudes

1. Compared to previous attempts, how motivated to lose weight are you this time?

1	2	3	4	5
Not at all motivated	Slightly motivated	Somewhat motivated	Quite motivated	Extremely motivated

2. How certain are you that you will stay committed to a weight loss program until you reach your goal?

1	2	3	4	5
Not at all certain	Slightly certain	Somewhat certain	Quite certain	Extremely certain

3. Consider all outside factors at this time (stress at work, family obligations, etc). To what extent can you tolerate the effort required to stick to a diet?

1	2	3	4	5
Cannot tolerate	Can tolerate somewhat	Uncertain	Can tolerate well	Can tolerate easily

4. Think honestly about how much weight you hope to lose and how quickly you hope to lose it. Figuring a weight loss of 1 to 2 pounds a week, how realistic is your expectation?

1	2	3	4	5
Very unrealistic	Somewhat unrealistic	Moderately unrealistic	Somewhat realistic	Very realistic

5. While dieting, do you fantasize about eating a lot of your favorite foods?

1	2	3	4	5
Always	Frequently	Occasionally	Rarely	Never

6. While dieting, do you feel deprived, angry, or upset?

1	2	3	4	5
Always	Frequently	Occasionally	Rarely	Never

Section 1: Total Score _____

If you scored:

6 to 16: This may not be a good time for you to start a weight loss program. Inadequate motivation and commitment, together with unrealistic goals, could block your progress. Think about those things that contribute to this, and consider changing them before undertaking a diet program.

17 to 23: You may be close to being ready to begin a program, but should think about ways to boost your preparedness before you begin.

24 to 30: The path is clear with respect to goals and attitudes.

Section 2: Hunger and Eating Cues

7. When food comes up in conversation or in something you read, do you want to eat even if you are not hungry?

1	2	3	4	5
Never	Rarely	Occasionally	Frequently	Always

8. How often do you eat because of physical hunger?

1	2	3	4	5
Always	Frequently	Occasionally	Rarely	Never

9. Do you have trouble controlling your eating when your favorite foods are around the house?

1	2	3	4	5
Never	Rarely	Occasionally	Frequently	Always

Section 2: Total Score _____

If you scored:

3 to 6: You might occasionally eat more than you would like, but it does not appear to result from high responsiveness to environmental cues. Controlling the attitudes that make you eat may be especially helpful.

7 to 9: You may have a moderate tendency to eat just because food is available. Dieting may be easier for you if you try to resist external cues and eat only when you are physically hungry.

10 to 15: Some or most of your eating may be in response to thinking about food or exposing yourself to temptations to eat. Think of ways to minimize your exposure to temptations so that you eat only in response to physical hunger.

Section 3: Control Over Eating

If the following situations occurred while you were on a diet, would you be likely to eat *more* or *less* immediately afterward and for the rest of the day?

10. Although you planned to skip lunch, a friend talks you into going out for a midday meal.

1	2	3	4	5
Would eat much less	Would eat somewhat less	Would make no difference	Would eat somewhat more	Would eat much more

11. You 'break' your diet by eating a fattening, 'forbidden' food.

1	2	3	4	5
Would eat much less	Would eat somewhat less	Would make no difference	Would eat some-what more	Would eat much more

12. You have been faithfully following your diet and decide to test yourself by eating something you consider a treat.

1	2	3	4	5
Would eat much less	Would eat somewhat less	Would make no difference	Would eat some-what more	Would eat much more

Section 3: Total Score _____

If you scored:

3 to 7: You recover rapidly from mistakes. However, if you frequently alternate between eating out of control and dieting very strictly, you may have a serious eating problem and should get professional help.

8 to 11: You do not seem to let unplanned eating disrupt your program. This is a flexible, balanced approach.

12 to 15: You may be prone to overeat after an event breaks your control or throws you off the track. Your reaction to these problem-causing eating events can be improved.

Section 4: Binge Eating and Purging

13. Aside from holiday feasts, have you ever eaten a large amount of food rapidly and felt afterward that this eating incident was excessive and out of control?

   2   Yes   0   No

14. If you answered yes to question 13, how often have you engaged in this behavior during the last year?

1	2	3	4	5	6
Less than once a month	About once a month	A few times a month	About once a week	About three times a week	Daily

15. Have you ever purged (used laxatives or diuretics, or induced vomiting) to control your weight?

5   Yes   0   No

16. If you answered yes to question 15, how often have you engaged in this behavior during the last year?

1	2	3	4	5	6
Less than once a month	About once a month	A few times a month	About once a week	About three times a week	Daily

Section 4: Total Score _____

If you scored:

0 to 1: It appears that binge eating and purging is not a problem for you.

2 to 11: Pay attention to these eating patterns. Get professional help if they arise more frequently.

12 to 19: You show signs of a potentially serious eating problem. See a counselor experienced in evaluating eating disorders right away.

Section 5: Emotional Eating

17. Do you eat more than you would like when you have negative feelings such as anxiety, depression, anger, or loneliness?

1	2	3	4	5
Never	Rarely	Occasionally	Frequently	Always

18. Do you have trouble controlling your eating when you have positive feelings—do you celebrate feeling good by eating?

1	2	3	4	5
Never	Rarely	Occasionally	Frequently	Always

19. When you have unpleasant interactions, or after a difficult day at work, do you eat more than you'd like?

1	2	3	4	5
Never	Rarely	Occasionally	Frequently	Always

Section 5: Total Score _____

If you scored:

3 to 8: You do not appear to let your emotions affect your eating.

9 to 11: You sometimes eat in response to emotional highs and lows. Monitor this behavior to learn when and why it occurs, and be prepared to find alternate activities.

12 to 15: Emotional ups and downs can stimulate your eating. Try to deal with the feelings that trigger the eating and find other ways to express them.

Section 6: Exercise Patterns and Attitudes

20. How often do you exercise?

1	2	3	4	5
Never	Rarely	Occasionally	Frequently	Always

21. How confident are you that you can exercise regularly?

1	2	3	4	5
Not at all confident	Slightly confident	Somewhat confident	Highly confident	Completely confident

22. When you think about exercise, do you develop a positive or negative picture in your mind?

1	2	3	4	5
Completely negative	Somewhat negative	Neutral	Somewhat positive	Completely positive

23. How certain are you that you can work regular exercise into your daily schedule?

1	2	3	4	5
Not at all certain	Slightly certain	Somewhat certain	Quite certain	Extremely certain

Section 6: Total Score _____

If you scored:

4 to 10: You're probably not exercising as regularly as you should. Determine whether your attitudes about exercise are blocking your way, then change what you must and put on those walking shoes.

11 to 16: You need to feel more positive about exercise so you can do it more often. Think of ways to be more active that are fun and fit your lifestyle.

17 to 20: It looks like the path is clear for you to be active.

After scoring yourself in each section of this questionnaire, you should be able to better judge your dieting strengths and weaknesses. Remember that the first step in changing eating behavior is to understand the conditions that influence your eating habits.

Appendix B

Guide for Behavior Change Toward Better Eating

Today you should begin to look at your eating patterns in a brand new way. The methods to increase awareness of eating behavior involve keeping detailed records of the food you eat. However, the end result is worth the effort.

Before we address how to keep these records, we focus on some of the basic goals of this diet plan, and present some facts about eating that will help you understand how to achieve them. *Changing your eating behavior* emphasizes new *learning* rather than specific diets.

The Behavior of Eating

- Eating is habitual; that is, it is done repeatedly and often without giving it much thought.
- Overweight, for many people, results from overeating; and overeating is often attributable to poor eating habits that have developed over long periods of time.
- Weight may be controlled by identifying these 'problem' habits and then changing them into new, more positive eating habits. The changes, therefore, can be permanent—a feature missing in crash diets that concentrate on including or eliminating specific foods rather than changing eating behavior.

- To make the change, you must first systematically observe and become aware of the specific habits that control your eating patterns. Then you can assume control over those problem areas. You may think you are aware of everything you eat now, but until you do it using the system we describe, you will not have a realistic picture of your eating behavior.

What is the Rationale of This Behavior Approach to Eating?

All behavior is produced by various cues or stimuli. Many stimuli may lead to eating, some of which are appropriate and some of which are not. For example, boredom, anxiety, depression, and the smell of food may be inappropriate stimuli for eating. Likewise, hunger, mealtimes, and certain social occasions are more appropriate stimuli. You must learn to *identify the appropriate stimuli* for eating, and also learn to substitute noneating activities for inappropriate stimuli.

You will discover the details of your own eating pattern: what, why, when, where, and how you eat. We examine each of these factors so you can become more fully aware of them.

How to Analyze Your Eating

- Remember, eating is behavior that is initiated by cues or triggers (stimuli) that lead to a response. This diagram shows these relationships.

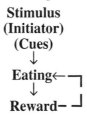

Stimulus
(Initiator)
(Cues)
↓
Eating←⌐
↓ |
Reward─⌐

- An association between each of these cues and the response of eating develops because, at some time, the stimulus was rewarded by eating. Although the initial rewards may no longer exist, the response of eating continues because of the earlier associations.
- To cite some examples: (1) The smell of food when you enter a house may trigger salivation and hunger. Eating satisfies the desire created by the smell of food. (2) If as a child you found that eating relieved feelings of anger or boredom, you would tend to eat again whenever you became angry or bored. (3) You may accept food offered at a party because you don't want to offend the hostess. Eating the food rewards you with the hostess' pleasure and appreciation, as well as a general feeling of social acceptance from the other guests.

Some cues or signals that may start or stop eating are listed below. The goal of this section is to determine which ones are important to you, and to help you control them.

- *Physiologic cues* include hunger, tension, growling stomach, headache, etc. Eating is an appropriate response to these stimuli.
- There are two kinds of *external cues*. The first are what we might call 'non-human.' They include the sight of food, smells of food, reading, watching television, and others. These cues are most easily identified and may be controlled by manipulating the events around us. The other external cues are 'human' in origin. They include the presence of friends, social events, coffee breaks, etc. These, too, can be controlled.
- *Emotional cues* like anger, depression, and boredom also can induce eating. These are often more difficult to control, but can be dealt with by changing the rewards and activities to which you respond.

Common Cues to Start Eating, With Recommended Responses

Physiologic Cues | **Suggested Controls (Examples)**

Growling stomach
Salivation
Faintness
Uneasy feeling
Headache
Hunger
Fatigue
Tension

The body produces these sensations when it expects or needs food. They are best controlled by always making it a habit to eat at a specific time. Establish a meal pattern, stick to it regularly, and these sensations eventually will appear only when it is *time to eat*, as planned. Make a ritual of where and when you eat. Substitute low-calorie food; keep prepared carrot sticks crisp and accessible for between meal snacks or appetizers when sensations of 'hunger' appear.

Bad taste in mouth (or other sensations)

Use mouthwash, toothpaste, or mouth spray.

External Cues (Non-human) | **Suggested Controls (Examples)**

Thoughts of food

Make yourself think of something else.

Shopping

Do it alone (friends and children increase the tendency to impulse shop). Always shop from a list. Never shop when hungry.

Cooking

Tell yourself the meal you are preparing is so great you don't want to spoil your appetite by nibbling. Choose low-calorie munchies or sip low-calorie

	drinks. If you train yourself to sit down to eat, it is harder to eat when cooking.
Smell of food	Use the same controls as for cooking (above). In a shopping center, plan to detour or avoid places emitting tempting odors.
Time of day (includes getting home from work, which may have some emotional cue component as well).	Stop to think whether you are truly hungry. Have a preplanned, pre-prepared, attractive meal or snack ready for quick service.
Weekends and holidays	Preplan your weekend eating. Holidays are associated with special meals; try to use controls, but enjoy the day.
Reading or other associated activities	Refer to discussion of associated activities.

External Cues (Human)

External Cues (Human)	**Suggested Controls (Examples)**
Others eating at meal times	Try to select, or prepare, low-calorie foods. Utilize built-in delays, as with other activities besides eating. Be the one to help the hostess.
Social events, parties, entertaining, etc	Do not stand or sit within easy reach of food. Avoid alcohol since even one drink can poison your control. At a cocktail party, try a drink made of soda and lemon juice; no one can tell it's not gin and tonic.

Emotional Cues	Suggested Controls (Examples)
Depression (includes feelings of failure) *Frustration* *Anger* *Boredom* *Lonely, unloved feelings* *Guilt* *Rebellion* *Feeling of deprivation*	These negative emotions are apparently common cues to start eating. However, they are 'down' attitudes and not generally helpful to self-image and self-motivation. Attempt to find and substitute other, more 'positive' cues. Develop a positive attitude— can be used in a cheerful, optimistic and self-motivating way.

Two groups of cues signal to stop eating. The following lists some of these, with suggestions for gaining control over internal and external signals.

Common Cues to Stop Eating, With Recommended Responses

Your goal is to develop new responses to strengthen and increase the frequency of cues that are already identified as 'stopping' eating, with emphasis on positive or appropriate types of controls rather than negative, inappropriate reactions.

Physiologic Cues	Suggested Controls (Examples)
Full (satisfied)	If only fullness stops your eating, you can never lose weight. Find or develop other cues to stop. If you don't know how, weigh food and eat to fullness. Next time, take a smaller portion.

Belt feels tight	Try tightening the belt one notch before beginning eating.
Drowsiness	A definite signal to stop eating immediately. You have no control when you are not fully alert and not concentrating.
Indigestion (discomfort)	This must be studied. Is it from pure overeating? Is it caused by certain foods or combination of foods? Does it occur when eating in association with something else (eg, certain mood, certain time of day, certain person)? First identify when and why discomfort occurs. Then, control the other associated factor.

External Cues (Nonhuman)

Food tastes bad	Very useful. You will practice how to increase your taste awareness later. Whenever you eat, be conscious of taste. If unpleasant, stop eating that food immediately. Food often begins to taste less good as you become physiologically satisfied. Therefore, changes in the taste of food should be a signal to stop eating.
Plate empty, ie, food all gone	Very common for most people. Demonstrates 'externality.' Can be used very positively to reduce food intake by choosing smaller plate, cooking only exact serving size, and eating slowly so you are not finished before others at table have ended their meal. Buying smaller amounts and shopping more often will also help.

Out of time (end of lunch hour) Something else you have to do	Become a calculating clock watcher and plan your activities. Example: At work, delay beginning of lunch hour meal by leisurely bathroom visit, stop to chat, a quick trip to bank, etc. Try to schedule other things to be done during problem-eating times. Commit yourself to trying alternate activities until you find one or more that suit you.

External Cues (Human)

Others at table	Slow eating to match pace of others at table. If you often eat with others, using this cue can really reduce total intake.

Emotional Cues

Feelings of achievement Satisfaction Happiness	Eating should be associated with good feelings, but, for weight control, other meaningful rewards must be used. Examples: pay yourself money, buy something special for yourself, call a friend to share the happiness, take a walk instead of eating.

Internal cues are physiologic, such as a full stomach, tight clothing, tight belt, and feelings of satiety. These are appropriate cues that we wish to attend to and respond to more rapidly.

A number of external cues also signal overeating. An empty plate is obvious. It is one of the most frequent, and is relatively easy to control. Next time, use a smaller plate, smaller portion sizes, and cook only what you can eat at one serving. Keeping serving dishes off the table can help control this type of cue. External cues can also come from human beings. These are usually different people or different circumstances than those that provide cues to start eating. However, we can capitalize on these to help stop eating earlier.

An understanding of these cues, and the exercise that follows, are designed to:

- help analyze your eating behavior and the specific signals that start and stop your eating
- control extraneous, irrelevant, or distorting stimuli by breaking their association with eating
- reinforce or reward new controls
- substitute other behavior for some eating incidents to control the frequency of eating
- make eating more pleasurable by becoming aware of the taste qualities of food
- increase your awareness of physical hunger as a cue to start and stop eating

Remember these behavior goals as you begin to identify the things you do when eating. Conscious awareness and self-observation is the key to controlling eating habits. Set short-term goals and stick to them.

For the next week, keep a record of what you do every time you eat, to learn what places are associated with your eating. This helps you identify those places that habitually cause you to eat.

You need an honest, current pattern of the things you do when you eat, so you can see how to control eating. These are for your benefit to help lose weight. Some changes may occur simply because you become more aware of what you are doing.

Eating and Where You Eat

Keeping Your Eating Record

The first exercise in analyzing your eating behavior involves identifying and then keeping a record of the places you eat. The techniques for making this analysis are used for all of the other evaluation exercises in the Physicians' Diet Plan. Thus, this section provides specific techniques to analyze your eating behavior in terms of what, when, why, and how you eat, so you may develop conscious control over all your eating activity.

During the coming week, pay attention to where you are every time you have something to eat. Watch for places that stimulate a desire to eat, such as walking past a bakery or a pizza parlor. Making a list may help you gain better control over the situations that trigger or stimulate eating.

Physicians' Diet Plan: Monitor for Places of Eating	
Day: _____	
Food Eaten	Place

This monitor card helps you keep a more detailed record of the places you eat each day. Keep your record for a full week. At the top of this monitor is a place to record the date or day of the week. Below it are two columns. On the left, write down the food you eat every time you put food in your mouth. Every bite of food—a cracker or a drink of anything except water—must be recorded. This means you must carry the monitor with you at all times. In the next column, write down the place where you ate the food. Because many people eat most of their food in only a few places, assigning numbers to the common places, like kitchen, dining room, den, cafeteria, etc, and then recording only the number, may be helpful.

The purpose of this monitor is to help you observe where you eat and to become more consciously *aware* of eating. The more accurate your records, the easier it will be to locate your problem areas and then change your eating habits. Be honest and thorough. You have only yourself to help! This is only the first of many records you will learn to keep. If you master it, the others will be easy. Use these guidelines to avoid possible pitfalls:

1. Remember to record everything you eat immediately.
   - Concentrate on eating and avoid other activities that can distract you.
   - Tying string on your finger may remind you of the record keeping.
   - Involve your spouse or a friend in the recording.
2. Keep your record even when you do not eat at home.
   - Have your monitor with you at all times; it is designed to fit into your pocket or purse.
   - If you prefer to make your recording privately, leave the table and record in the privacy of the bathroom.
3. Learn to identify what goes into the food you eat.
   - Concentrate on the food and examine what you eat. This is part of the goal of becoming more aware of your eating behavior.
   - At a friend's house, request the recipe; the cook will be flattered.
   - At restaurants, people who are on special diets (eg, diabetics) often request information on ingredients. Play allergic, if necessary.

A Week Passes

Analyzing the Record of Where You Eat

During the past week, you recorded what you ate and where you ate it. This week you will learn how to analyze these records and recognize your patterns of eating. You may find you need to reduce the number of places you eat.

Look at the monitors you have used during the past week. Below is an illustration of a completed analysis for places of eating to show you what the finished result might look like. Several places where people commonly eat are printed, and several empty lines have been left for your use.

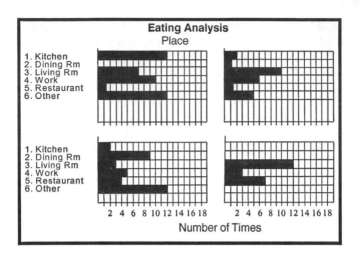

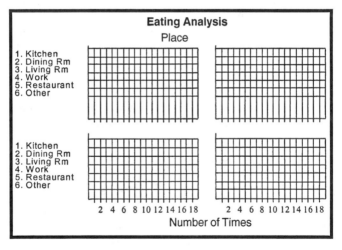

First, add the places you ate that are not listed on the form. Next, blacken a box opposite the first place you ate on day 1. For example, if you ate breakfast in the kitchen, lunch in a restaurant, a snack in your office, dinner in the dining room, and a snack in the kitchen, then your form should contain two black squares for kitchen, one blackened square for dining room, one for work, and one for restaurants. Continue to fill in the places you ate until all 7 days have been transferred to the analysis sheet.

How an Awareness of Where You Eat Can Help You Control Eating

- Certain places often become, by habit of long association, direct stimuli to eat. They may include ball games, movies, or a chair by the television.
- Some people eat everywhere and anywhere. Instead of saying, "I can't eat," tell yourself, "I can eat only in one or two designated places."
- Eliminate first the places not directly associated with food. However, be flexible. For example, if you live in an efficiency apartment, it may not be possible to stop eating in the bedroom. However, you don't have to eat in bed!
- Making a big occasion of each eating incident may be helpful. Set a place at your own designated eating area, use special dishes, a special place mat, flowers or candles, etc.
- You may want to designate one special place to eat at home (and also one at work) and simply change the habit of where you eat. Eating only at that place may help you gain control.
- Eating in the cafeteria at work is appropriate. Eating at your desk or elsewhere is inappropriate. Circle these inappropriate times on your analysis sheet and try to stop eating at your desk. Move to the cafeteria or a different part of the office to eat.
- Your goal is to reduce the number of places you eat.

You are now ready to repeat the monitoring for another week to see how successful you have been in changing the number of places you eat. Complete a second analysis form in the same way.

Eating and Its Associated Activities
Monitoring Your Eating and Activities

This section is designed to help you become aware of the things you do while you eat. Remember, eating is a behavior that can be initiated by both internal and external cues or stimuli. The need to eat is inborn, but culture teaches us to adapt this need in accepted ways. In our culture, rewards are often associated with food. Positive rewards tend to strengthen the association between eating behavior and the cues that lead to it. Negative rewards tend to weaken these associations.

Physicians' Diet Plan: Monitor for Associated Activity	
Day: ____	
Food Eaten	Associated Activity

The goal of this monitor is to help you focus on the problem areas associated with eating and make step-by-step changes to achieve gradual control. Remember, the more accurate your records, the more they will ultimately help you change your patterns. You will see a box for the day at the top of the form. Fill it in for that day. You may use numbers (Day 1, Day 2, etc) or abbreviations (M, Tu, W, Th).

In column 1, write down the foods you eat. Recording every bite and every sip you put in your mouth is essential, including low or noncalorie foods and drinks. Record immediately as you eat. If you do not have your monitor with you, it is better to not record that food or meal at all. Never fill in the monitor from memory. Inaccurate records are misleading.

In the column on the right, record what you are doing when eating. For example, at lunch, you are eating at the dining room table at a friend's house, and you are talking. You should record food eaten (such as a fruit salad, soup, and coffee) and the fact that you were talking with your friend.

The most common activities associated with eating are watching television, talking, reading, and preparing food. You may want to give these activities numbers (1-4) and only write the other things you do while eating. Keep your record for a full week on the set of monitors.

A Week Passes

Analyzing Your Eating and Its Associated Activities

Now that you have a week's record of the activities associated with your eating behavior, you are ready to analyze them. Below is an illustration of what an analysis form might look like.

Physicians' Diet Plan: Analysis of Associated Activity

	1	2	3	4	5	6	7	8	9	10	11	12	13	14	Add'l	Total
Reading	■	■	■	■	■											5
Watching TV	■	■	■													3
Preparing Meal	■	•														2
Talking	■	■	■													3
None	■	■	■	■												4
Other																
Other	■	■														2

Physicians' Diet Plan: Analysis of Associated Activity

	1	2	3	4	5	6	7	8	9	10	11	12	13	14	Add'l	Total
Reading																
Watching TV																
Preparing Meal																
Talking																
None																
Other																
Other																

Begin by assembling the monitor cards you used this past week. Notice, on the analysis form, that the four most common activities associated with eating (reading, watching television, preparing food, talking) are listed. Blank spaces can contain any other activities you did while eating. Fill in a square, beginning at the left, for each instance of eating at the appropriate activity. Do this for the entire week, blackening one square for every time you had something to eat.

Use the column labeled 'additional' (add'l) for any number of events over 14. This can be done by putting extra check marks in this box to indicate each extra instance of eating. Circle the square if that eating instance consisted only of noncaloric food, such as black coffee, tea, or diet soda. If the beverage had sugar or milk in it, or if anything else was consumed, do not circle it.

When you have gone through the entire week's records, count the number of checks and boxes and put the total number in the last column, labeled total.

Awareness of Associated Activities Can Be Used To Control Eating

Associated activities, like places of eating, can become cues for eating. An awareness of activity is important because research has shown that overweight people eat more when they are distracted. It is easy to overeat when you are engrossed in a book, television, or conversation. When people do not pay attention to food and eating, they cannot use conscious controls. The eating is done automatically and unconsciously.

The following guidelines can help you:

- Make a conscious effort to turn off the television and avoid reading when you eat. Your goal is to make eating enjoyable in itself. Distracting events may lead you to eat more than you otherwise would.
- We don't advise 'no talking when eating,' as pleasant sociability while eating may be important. However, take your mind off the conversation every minute or two to concentrate upon your food and your feelings about it. Concentrate on how you eat: slowly, chewing thoroughly, savoring the flavors. All this means that whenever you eat, you should try to do little else.
- Your goal is to reduce noneating activities associated with eating, while enjoying your food more fully.

Substitute Alternative Behavior

A number of cues or signals may automatically trigger eating, but you can change these patterns. Some added suggestions:

1. Television food commercials
   - Change channels.
   - Leave the room (this also increases exercise).
   - Do a self-rewarding chore or activity (eg, wash a shelf, change clothing, brush teeth).
   - Try to reduce television time, especially if associated with eating.

2. Sight of food
   - Keep food out of sight.
   - Use opaque containers.
   - Repackage food as soon as you bring it home from the market.
   - Don't put serving containers on the table; put portions directly on plates.
   - Remove leftovers immediately and scrape plates into disposal.
3. Thought of food
   - Try not to think about food; put it out of your mind by thinking about something else. This is a substitute activity, replacing one thought for another.
4. Change the way you eat
   - Choose low-calorie foods over high-calorie foods.
   - Build in delays in the rate of eating. For example, drink water between bites or go to the powder room. Help in serving or clearing food as a substitute activity.
5. Emotional cues
   - Eating is not an appropriate response to emotional situations. Develop substitute activities for boredom or depression, such as taking a hot bath, walking, reading, involving yourself with a hobby, or calling a friend. Eating is not an appropriate response to anger or guilt. Physical exercise often helps relieve this kind of tension. Emotions, in general, are arousing. This means that happy emotions, as well as anger and depression, can trigger overeating. Therefore, it is important to learn appropriate responses to emotions, as well as knowing which cues and activities may trigger your eating.

After completing the week's analysis of activities associated with eating, you can apply what you have learned by recording these activities for a second week, using some of the controls and behavior changes we have discussed.

Eating and Hunger
Monitoring Eating and Hunger

The third monitor is for your personal evaluation of hunger; that is, how hungry you are every time you have something to eat. These questions may be helpful:

1. What is hunger?
2. How do you experience hunger?

The following are some of the answers we have had from patients. Which ones do you associate with hunger?

salivation	tension	lightheadedness
growling	knots in stomach	weakness
depression	nausea	irritability
headache	anxiety	'climbing the wall'

3. How hungry are you right now? Very hungry, not hungry, somewhat hungry?
4. How often do you eat when you are not really hungry?

When filling out this monitor, we want you to be able to distinguish between the physical sensations of hunger and the desire to eat. Appetite and hunger are different. *Appetite* refers to a *desire for food*, often for a particular food. *Hunger* indicates a *physiologic need for food*.

During the coming week, you will use this monitor for evaluating hunger to record your hunger at the beginning of each meal.

- Focus on how hungry you are as you start each eating incident.
- Note whether it is a full meal or a snack.
- Each time you start to eat (a meal or a snack), take a moment to decide how hungry you are.

    Use a rating scale of 1 to 5, as follows:

    1 = no hunger
    2 = slightly hungry
    3 = moderately hungry
    4 = very hungry
    5 = extremely hungry

Define hunger as you sense it. Note the different sensations of hunger, if any.

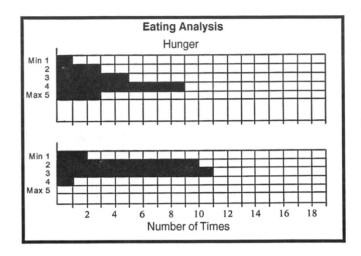

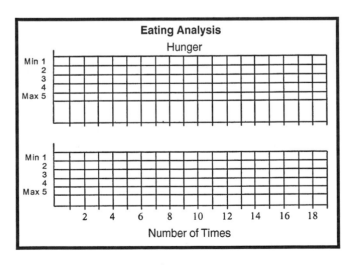

A Week Passes

Analyzing Your Hunger Ratings

Now that you have recorded your relative hunger during 1 week, you are ready to analyze how this relates to your eating behavior. A sample of what a finished analysis form might look like is shown above.

The hunger ratings (1 to 5) are printed in the left column; the number of times you recorded each rating for the past week are printed across the bottom. Fill in the form as you did before:

- Mark a square beside the appropriate hunger rating for each time you felt that degree of hunger.
- Use check marks for any additional ratings at each level.
- Count all boxes plus additional checks and record the total number of each rating.
- Circle any noncaloric food.

Hunger is an internal tension that may be perceived as headaches, depression, anxiety, or a growling sensation. Your goal is to become more responsive to your body's signals of hunger. Two factors should be considered:

1. Are you finding it easier to identify hunger? If not, keep practicing until you can separate physiologic sensations from environmental cues.
2. When are you hungry? Some people find it easy to identify hunger patterns; others find it hard. It may help to rearrange your meal schedule to eat when you are hungry; when you identify cues other than true hunger, try to do something other than eat. This is where hobbies and other activities you enjoy are particularly important.

You can begin to control your behavior based on responses to hunger *while* eating. For the coming week, at one meal each day, stop eating as soon as you realize you are no longer hungry. Select and write down at *which* meal each day you will practice that response (select the meal most regularly included in your daily pattern).

Your goal is to learn to 'tune in' to your body signals to better understand personal hunger and recognize the cues that trigger your appetite. These are some of the results you may expect:

1. Your attitude toward your food may change. Leave waste on the plate, not on your waist. When parents taught that waste is 'sinful,' you were being trained to overeat. However, eating more than you need is also wasting food. A little wasting (or discarding) of food now can be compensated for later as you learn to shop and eat more economically.

2. You may consider not eating dessert. This might mean taking more food than planned (in second helpings) to stop the feeling of hunger and the urge to eat the wrong foods.

For the coming week, ask yourself how hungry you are before a meal or snack, and try to eliminate as many ratings in the #1 and #2 columns as you can. You don't have to be ravenous (#5), but try to be moderately hungry before eating (#3 and #4). This may mean skipping a meal if you decide that you are not really hungry at that time.

Eating and the Taste of Food

Taste is a subjective valuation that elicits different responses from different people. Ask yourself what taste means to you. Is there a *good* taste? A *bad* taste? How do you taste food? Some of the factors that determine sense of taste include flavor, aroma, and texture. You may gain better control over eating habits by improving your perception of taste.

Try the following tests with some dehydrated apple slices and some flavored crackers:

- Unwrap the package of dried apples very slowly. Is your mouth watering? If it is, you know that external cues (eg, the thought, smell, and sight of food) are triggering your hunger. This can be a very strong incentive to eat.

- Take a slice of apple, but do not start eating. Look at the apple. Smell it. What sensation do you feel?
- Take a small bite, but don't swallow. Chew it thoroughly and slowly. How does it taste?
- Continue to chew slowly. Does the taste change? How?
- Now, repeat the steps with the crackers. First, open the package as slowly as you can. Is your mouth watering?
- Take a cracker, but do not start eating. Look at it, smell it. What do you feel?
- Take a small bite, but don't swallow. Chew it slowly and thoroughly. Try to taste it as intensely as you can. How does it taste? Do the taste and texture change as you continue to chew the cracker?
- What does this test really tell you about tasting food?
- You must chew your food thoroughly.
- Decide how good a food tastes by judging how long-lasting its flavor is.

Flavors change with enzyme action in saliva, but you won't notice that if you gulp down your food. Appearance, smell, and texture influence the sensation of taste. From now on, try to really practice tasting everything you eat, just as you did with the apples and crackers.

Recording the Taste of Food

For the next week, your record-keeping will focus on the taste of your food. A sample of the taste monitor is shown below.

Write down on the left every mouthful of food you eat at the time you eat it. As you put the food into your mouth, do what you have just done with the dried apples and crackers. That is, let the food stay in your mouth for a few seconds, and then chew it slowly. Evaluate the taste on a scale of 1 to 5. Use the following rating scale:

Physicians' Diet Plan: Monitor for Taste	
Day: _____	
Food Eaten	Taste of Food

1 = tastes poorly or no taste
2 = taste is fair
3 = good-tasting
4 = very good taste
5 = fantastic taste

Do this with each different food item. Note and record how taste changes as you go through the meal bite after bite. Do you keep eating after the flavor changes? If so, here may be the opportunity for you to make some changes. Keep this record for 1 week.

A Week Passes

Analyzing Your Eating and the Taste of Food

Now that you have recorded how you taste food for a full week, you can begin to analyze how taste affects your eating habits. A sample taste analysis form is reproduced below, which is similar to the other forms we have used.

On the left side are taste ratings (1 to 5); across the top are the number of times you recorded each rating during the past week. Count your ratings and fill in the squares as you did when rating hunger. Circle any noncaloric foods.

Your goal with this monitor is to heighten taste awareness and enjoyment of food.

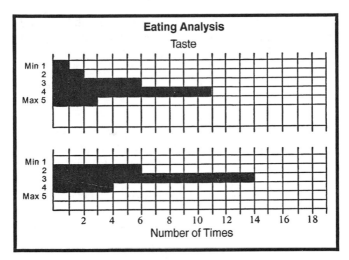

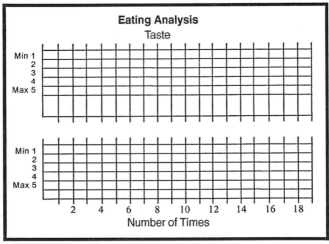

In the coming week, try to increase the number of ratings in columns #3 and #4, and reduce the number of ratings in columns #1 and #2. Too many #5 ratings can stimulate overeating.

For the next week, repeat the monitoring of the taste of your foods.

Further Analysis of Eating and the Taste of Foods

As you did last week, record all your taste ratings from everything you ate. Follow the same procedure, always beginning at the left.

Were you able to make changes? What were they? How did you do it? Continue to evaluate the taste of your food when you are hungry and after you are full. Remember, awareness can give you control over eating.

- Any time you realize you are no longer hungry, stop eating.
- Any time you are not really hungry, don't eat.
- Anything not tasting good (#3, #4, or #5) should lead you to ask yourself 'why am I eating this?'

Your goal is to break the cue-response chains that help you retain bad eating habits. Several techniques can help you change your habits:

1. Select a specific place to do all your eating.
2. Eat on one special plate of small size, with your own special utensils.
3. Always sit down to eat. This makes it difficult to nibble while preparing food or doing other activities.
4. Eliminate distracting influences while eating, such as reading or watching television.
5. Try to internalize and personalize these ideas so they apply to your needs and problems.
6. Do not try to eliminate your most difficult problems first. 'Cut down rather than cut out' should be your motto for the early changes.

Frequency and Rate of Eating

How *fast* and how *often* you eat are two important factors that affect your overall eating behavior. Learning about the *frequency* and *rate* of eating help you identify problem areas and change more positive habits. The monitor is shown below.

Physicians' Diet Plan: Monitor for Frequency and Rate of Eating			
Day: _____			
Food Eaten	Time		Meal or Snack
	Start	Stop	

In column #1, list all the foods and beverages you eat, just as with the previous monitors for where you eat and for the associated activities. Remember, you must record immediately each time you eat. Do not rely on memory; carry the monitors with you at all times.

Under the column 'Time-Start', write down the *exact time* (eg, 10:16, 12:21) when you start eating anything, even one bite. You must have a clock or watch available at all times. You must also have your monitor available at all times. Don't rely on memory. To see why this is important, try to recall how many separate times you ate yesterday. What time did each incident start; when did it stop? You can see how difficult it is to remember these things even 1 day later.

In the column 'Time-Stop', record the exact time you stopped eating each meal or snack. In the second column, 'Meal or Snack', write 'M' for meal or 'S' for snack. Spend the next 7 days recording frequency and timing of your meals and snacks.

A Week Passes

Analysis for the Frequency of Eating

A completed sample of each is shown below.

The left column for frequency analysis divides the day into 1-hour periods. Across the top is the number of eating incidents. From your monitor cards, count the number of meals and snacks. Each incident should be recorded separately. Fill in or mark the number of squares for that time period, 1 day at a time. Mark the time column when you began to eat. Circle each noncaloric (eg, black cof-

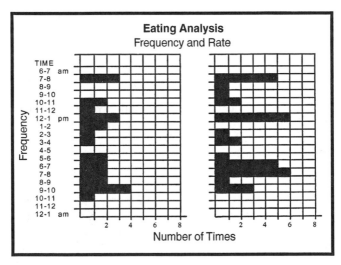

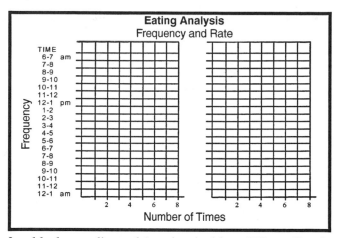

fee, black tea, diet soda) eating incident. When all columns are filled in, use marks in the 'additional' column. Put the total number in the 'total' column.

Analysis for the Rate of Eating

The left side of the rate analysis has the number of minutes for each eating incident. Across the top is the number

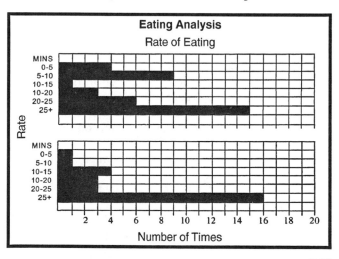

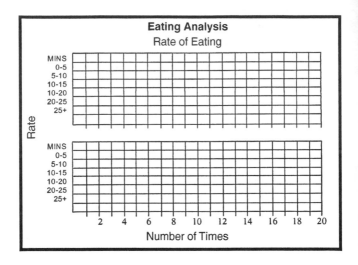

Eating Analysis
Rate of Eating

MINS
0-5
5-10
10-15
10-20
20-25
25+

Rate

MINS
0-5
5-10
10-15
10-20
20-25
25+

2   4   6   8   10   12   14   16   18   20
Number of Times

of eating occasions. Count the number of minutes spent on each meal or snack. Fill in the squares for the number of eating occasions beside each time period. Remember to circle each noncaloric eating incident.

Controlling the Frequency of Eating
1. If your problem is eating all day long, you can control it by reducing the number of times you eat.
    *   Preplanning and pre-preparing can be a good defense strategy. When you get up in the morning, plan when and where you will eat that day. This will help control your responses to those food-associated stimuli that can turn you 'on' at any particular moment.
    *   Eat only when and what you planned.
    *   Select a 1-hour period when you will eat nothing. Pick an hour that has at least one eating instance a week that is not a meal.
    *   Try to control where you eat and the activities associated with eating. As you change one, other as-

pects will be affected. The results from the behavior change will be multiplied with every small change.

- Do not attempt to eat much food at meals or at breakfast to reduce the number of other instances. Cut out, but do not replace.

2. If your problem is eating most of your food at meal times, try other tactics:

- Use a smaller plate; portions will look larger.
- Do not put serving dishes on the table. This makes it harder to get second helpings.
- Eat more slowly. This gives you a chance to feel full earlier. When others at the table are done, stop, even if food is left on your plate.
- Have sparkling water with ice and lemon juice or a diet drink before meals.
- If you have a three-meal pattern, determine if that includes everything you ate. If it does, your problem may not be the frequency but the quantity eaten at each meal.

Controlling the Rate of Eating

1. If most meals are eaten in 10 minutes or less, the body's signals for satiety may not have time to tell you to stop. The food may not have time to signal you that you've had enough by activating internal responses.

- Aim for 10 to 25 minutes for each meal.
- Sit down to eat all meals.
- Concentrate on enjoying food by having an attractive table setting, using nice dishes, and trying to really taste your food. This requires chewing thoroughly.
- Do not drink liquid except when your mouth is empty.
- Plan occasional 1- to 2-minute delays between courses.

- Do not put serving dishes on the table (to reduce ease of second helpings).
- Pause between bites. Cut food into smaller pieces. Try to chew more slowly. This gives you a chance to feel full.
- In a restaurant, watch thin people eat. They often put down utensils between bites, wipe their mouths, etc. All of this slows down the eating process.

2. Liquids can be an important control mechanism.
- Liquids can increase the volume of the stomach, helping to signal that you've had enough to eat.
- Drink one or more glasses of water a meal.
- Learn to put down your knife and fork between bites. Concentrate on building in delays. Drink water between finishing one bite and taking the next.
- As noted before, some fast eaters wash down unchewed food. The emphasis should be on changing rapid eating (5 minutes or less) and prolonged eating (over 26 minutes).
- Try to keep more eating events toward the middle (10 to 25 minutes). Again, remember to make simple, gradual changes.

Preplanning

Preplanning Meals

The goal is to begin preplanning and begin to focus on practical ways to control your eating. The technique includes an analysis form in which the kinds of activity that were preplanned and executed can be recorded. This tool prepares you for difficult situations: meals away from home, foods eaten during the weekend, parties, and other social occasions where temptation to overeat may be a problem.

In the coming week, pick a time to try preplanning. There are three assignments.

Physicians' Diet Plan: Preplanning	
Activity Preplanned	

Physicians' Diet Plan: Preplanning	
Recording Side for Preplanned Day	

For two days, a 'regular,' routine day, and a 'weekend' day, preplan one part of the day. Choose from the following what you are going to eat, the amounts you think you will eat, the exact time you will eat, or where you will eat. Do this the evening before or the first thing in the morning on that day. Make sure it is not done at the very last moment. The goal is to enable you to make conscious decisions about what, when, where, and how much you eat. Also, remember that changes in your activities may require you to alter them.

On the selected day, record what you actually ate, including the exact time and amounts. This gives you a chance to apply awareness of calories and of eating situations, and restructure your plan if circumstances change.

For example: friends invite you to a restaurant for dinner. Before going, think about what you will order. This insulates you against the psychologic turn-on most of us experience when presented with a menu and its many choices.

If your plan fails, you can still get useful information from it. Analyze and write down why you were unable to follow the plan. Then, rather than blaming yourself or anyone else, try to develop a plan once again.

A Week Passes

Analysis of Preplanning

During the past week, you have preplanned 1 meal or 1 day. How did it go?

For how many days did you preplan and then record actual intake?

The goals of preplanning are:
- to help you identify difficult situations before they arise
- to help you make a more conscious approach to these difficult situations
- to give you the upper hand by planning ahead rather than becoming a victim of fate

How accurate was your preplanning? Record on the chart your answers to the questions on the form below.

For each day or part of a day that you preplanned, record whether you ate or didn't eat what you planned. Also record whether you ate more or less than you planned. In the Physicians' Maintenance Plan, we return to planning and solving difficult eating situations.

Physicians' Diet Plan
Analysis of Preplanning
Number of Times

	Number of Times													
	1	2	3	4	5	6	7	8	9	10	11	12	Add'l	Total
Food item eaten not planned														
Food item planned not eaten														
More food eaten than planned														
Less food eaten than planned														
Eating at time/place not planned														
Ate as planned (Gold Star)														

Physicians' Diet Plan
Analysis of Preplanning
Number of Times

	Number of Times													
	1	2	3	4	5	6	7	8	9	10	11	12	Add'l	Total
Food item eaten not planned	■													
Food item planned not eaten	■	■												
More food eaten than planned	■													
Less food eaten than planned														
Eating at time/place not planned	■													
Ate as planned (Gold Star)	■	■	■											

Preplanning can have several uses:
- It can help with planning *weekends*.
- It can be used when dining out. Although you cannot anticipate what the hostess will serve, you *can* plan what to cut down on, how to leave food on your plate,

how to praise the dessert but not finish it, and how to win support for your weight goals from others by showing proper restraint.

Some helpful tips include drinking plenty of water, using the bathroom during the dinner hour to delay the rate of eating, and putting your fork down between each bite. Because alcohol dulls your taste and ability to follow your plan, avoid alcoholic drinks if possible.

The same method can help you in:

- planning for business luncheons
- planning for holidays or trips
- planning for days when emotional problems are apt to arise (report cards, end of the month bills, etc)
- planning for shopping trips

Appendix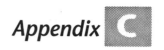

Guide To Better Nutrition

Why must we eat? *What* should we eat? The answers to these questions are what nutrition is all about.

Food contains more than 40 nutrients that the body needs in proper amounts to function. The nutrients are water, oxygen, proteins, carbohydrates, fat, vitamins, and minerals. The carbohydrate, fat, and, to a lesser extent, protein, provide the energy we use every day.

From these nutrients, the body prepares the thousands of substances needed to maintain life and provide physical stamina, mental alertness, emotional stability, and energy. *Good nutritional habits* are essential to maintaining good health.

Being *overweight* does not necessarily mean you are *well nourished*. It is quite possible to be *poorly nourished* and yet *overweight* at the same time.

In overweight, only the *number* or *amount* of calories is involved. If your only concern is losing weight, then all you have to do is reduce or eliminate calories. If you want to be healthy as well, there are other concerns:

- To maintain good health, you must *meet the nutritional needs* of your body.
- To maintain an acceptable weight, you must find *well-balanced* yet *palatable* foods that suit your own likes and dislikes.

Thus, an individual eating plan must have both the correct number of calories and the correct type of foods, including preferred foods.

You can make individual choices within these limits. We want to help you understand how to use these limits.

To start, let's see how much you know about nutrition. The questions below cover some of the basic knowledge on nutrition, and will be answered. Meanwhile, see how well you do on this initial nutrition assessment.

Your Nutrition Quotient

Instructions: Matching Test

Select the letter of the word or phrase in Column II that best describes or defines each item in Column I. Write that letter (a, b, c, etc) on the blank line.

Column I	Column II
1. The main nutrient in milk that makes it indispensable in human diets _____	a. Protein
	b. Starch
	c. Saturated fat
2. Building blocks of proteins _____	d. Dextrose
	e. Fiber
3. Main type of fat in corn oil _____	f. Calcium
	g. Vitamin C
4. Vitamin in strawberries _____	h. Cholesterol
5. Cellulose _____	i. Water
6. Main component of human body _____	j. Calorie
	k. Amino acids
7. A measure of heat _____	l. Vitamin B
8. The main nutrient in meat _____	m. None of the above

Instructions: Multiple-Choice Test

Select the best answer for each question and circle the letter.

9. A pound of human fat contains _____ calories.
   a. 1,500 b. 2,500 c. 3,500 d. 4,500 e. 5,500

10. The basal metabolism of men is _____ that of women.
    a. same as   b. higher than   c. lower than

11. A major source of vitamin C is _____.
    a. liver   b. green vegetables   c. citrus fruits
    d. lean meats   e. bread & grains

12. Vegetable fats are usually _____.
    a. saturated fats low in cholesterol
    b. unsaturated fats low in cholesterol
    c. saturated fats high in cholesterol
    d. unsaturated fats high in cholesterol

13. Fiber in the diet is mainly _____.
    a. carbohydrate   b. protein   c. fat   d. water

The three types of 'fuel' or food energy provided by food are contained in the:
    1. carbohydrates
    2. proteins
    3. fats

We will define each in turn, describing the type of foods that contain them and their function in the body.

We will also tell you how to use this information to prepare your own well-balanced, healthy, and delicious calorie-controlled food plan for optimum health. We call this food plan the *Menumax*® Meal Planner because it maximizes your nutrition in the menus you plan.

Calories

The human body has a delicate energy balance. In nutrition, energy is measured in calories. The body needs this energy, or calories, to do all of its work, such as movement, digestion, making cells, destroying cells, removing wastes, breathing, circulating the blood, etc.

Energy is measured as calories. A calorie is the amount of heat required to raise 1 g of water 1 degree centigrade (from 15 to 16 degrees). The caloric values of food tell us the amount of energy or heat the body gets when that food is used in the body.

Daily calorie needs change:
- They decline with age.
- They increase with body size and weight.
- They are higher in men than in women at the same age, height, and weight.
- They are modified by glandular function.

Most adults require between 1,500 and 3,500 calories a day. The National Academy of Sciences estimates that an average 64" female, age 19-22, weighing 120 lb (55 kg), needs 2,100 calories a day. The average male, 70", age 19-22, weighing 154 lb (70 kg), needs 2,900 calories a day.

The energy stored as fat in fatty tissue contains 3,500 calories in each pound. To lose 1 pound of body fat, you must use 3,500 calories more than you eat.

During one year, we eat between 700,000 and 1,000,000 calories, depending on size, sex, and age. Storing as fat only 1% of those calories, that is, 7,000 to 10,000 calories, can result in a weight gain of 2 to 3 pounds each year.

Let's examine what happens if we eat and store 100 calories more each day than we burn. The following are foods with approximately 100 calories:
- Apple, 2" diameter
- Applesauce, 1 cup unsweetened
- Bacon, 2 slices, fried crisp
- Butter, 1 T
- Hershey's milk chocolate bar, without nuts, 2/3 oz
- Pepsi-Cola, 8 oz
- Cookies: 2 chocolate chip (commercial), 6 ginger snaps, 6 vanilla wafers
- Green beans, fresh, 3 1/4 cups
- Ham, fresh, lean, marbled, cooked, 1 1/2 oz
- Roast chicken: light meat without skin or bones, 2 oz

An extra 100 calories more than we use each day for 35 days results in a weight gain of 1 pound as stored fat. If this continues, ie, if 100 calories a day are stored as fat, you will gain 10 pounds a year, or 100 pounds in 10 years!

Because any method of treating overweight must either decrease calorie intake, increase calorie output, or both, we could simply eat less, and exercise more. However, this is easier said than done. We know that 'wild' animals seem to keep their body weight constant with a balanced storage of energy. They eat only when fuel is needed (hungry). Intuitively, they know that otherwise they might become less agile and end up as another animal's dinner.

With 'civilization' and changes in our ways of living, humans now eat for reasons other than the simple need for food. Thus, to control calories one must both directly focus on them, as we are doing here, or indirectly focus on where, when, and how one eats.

To lose weight permanently, you must reduce the amount of stored energy. You can control two factors on the diagram of energy balance (page D-1): *Food Intake* and *Exercise* or *Movement*.

To recapitulate: to lose weight, you must decrease caloric *intake* or increase caloric *output*. If you need 1,800 calories a day and you take in 1,300 calories a day, there is a deficit of 500 calories a day. Over 7 days, this equals 3,500 calories or the equivalent of 1 pound a week of weight loss as fat.

If your caloric intake is 1,000 calories/day less than you need for a week, you can expect to lose 2 pounds (7,000 calories) of fat from fat tissue in a week.

Fluctuations in the amount of water in the body can increase or decrease this weight loss. It is important to keep in mind that when the body burns up fat, it produces water. To lose weight from burning up fat, we must excrete the water. *The weight of the water produced by burning fat weighs more than the fat that is burned.* Thus, for short periods of time, you can eat fewer calories than you need and yet gain weight from the water formed during the use (metabolism) of this fat. But don't be discouraged: this is a *short-term* process and, eventually, the body will excrete this extra water and you will be lighter.

Physicians' Diet Plan: Monitor for Calories			
Day: _____			
Food Eaten	Amount (Weight)	Calories	
		Solid	Liquid

Maintaining the Calories You Eat in Food

We will use a monitor to record the calories you eat, similar to the one shown in the sample above. Each time you eat, including every meal and every snack, write down the food eaten.

Also write down, as accurately as possible, the amount eaten. Use whatever measurement is most familiar to you. Aim for the greatest possible accuracy. At the earliest opportunity, and at least once a day, look up the number of calories in the amount of each food you ate.

A number of books list caloric content of foods. Lists are available in your bookstore. Almost all lists are based on one of two sources: (1) The U.S. Department of Agriculture *Handbook No. 8, Composition of Foods: Raw, Processed, Prepared*; or (2) Bowes and Church: *Food Values of Portions Commonly Used* (J.B. Lippincott Co). The book by B. Kraus, *Calories and Carbohydrates* (Grosset and Dunlap), a dictionary to 7,500 brand names and basic foods with calorie and carbohydrate counts, is particularly useful because it contains information on many packaged foods.

Record the calories under liquid or solid. When you have completed the eight calorie monitors shown in the book, you will be ready to evaluate your calorie intake.

Physicians' Diet Plan: Analysis of Caloric Intake

	Daily Total							
	1	2	3	4	5	6	7	Grand Total
Solid								
Liquid								
Sum								

Physicians' Diet Plan: Analysis of Caloric Intake

	Daily Total							
	1	2	3	4	5	6	7	Grand Total
Solid	1200	1000	1500	1450	1550	1000	1250	8950
Liquid	200	150	300	100	150	100	150	1150
Sum	1400	1150	1800	1550	1700	1100	1400	10,100

A Week Passes

Analysis of Caloric Intake

Now that you have recorded your caloric intake and the foods you have eaten for the past week, it is time to analyze the results. Place your calorie monitor in front of you.

Step 1: Add up total caloric intake ingested as liquids for Day 1. Record that total in the column marked 'Liquid' on the line for Day 1.

Step 2: Add up total caloric intake for the solid food eaten on Day 1. Record this total under 'Solids' on Day 1.

Step 3: Repeat above steps for each of the 7 days of your monitors.

Step 4: On the far right lines, record the daily caloric intake by adding Liquids and Solids for each day.

Some key points:

Calorie totals may appear surprisingly low. Many people don't seem to need much food because they are relatively inactive. There is also a wide variation from day to day. This indicates a need for greater awareness for preplanning to help better control your eating. This also reemphasizes the importance of response to external stimuli.

A high calorie intake as liquid may signify a 'problem' liquid. Soft drinks and alcoholic beverages are the usual culprits.

If totals are below 1,000-1,200, you are probably losing weight. If not, you may need a careful way of measuring the amounts of food or more diligence in recording every time you eat. Accurate caloric values in foods are difficult to obtain for several reasons.

- Estimates of portion sizes often are inaccurate.
- Food combinations can be difficult to estimate unless a package label lists calories.
- The caloric contents of food from restaurants and cafeterias can be difficult to obtain. When in doubt, pick a higher amount.

Helpful Tools to Monitor Your Food

We have already described one way of monitoring your calorie intake. Other ways can make calorie counting simpler and more fun: nutrition labels, the measuring cup, calorie scale, and food models.

Nutrition Labels

Nutrition labels on canned and packaged foods are an important outgrowth of the efforts of nutritionists on behalf of consumers. Any food in the grocery store advertised as having 'nutritional value' must have a nutrition label. One example of this format is shown (low-fat milk). This food was selected for two reasons. First, it shows the nature of the nutrition label on all foods. Second, it showcases the use of the low-fat label, which means a reduction of more than 50% over the natural food. In reduced-

LOWFAT MILK

NUTRITION FACTS

Serving Size 8 fl oz (240 ml)
Servings Per Container 8

Amount per Serving

Calories 100   Calories from Fat 20

	%Daily Value*
Total Fat 2.5g	4%
Saturated Fat 1.5g	8%
Cholesterol 10mg	3%
Sodium 130mg	5%
Total Carbohydrate 12g	4%
Dietary Fiber 0g	0%
Sugars 11g	
Protein 8g	

Vitamin A 10g	•	Vitamin C 4%
Calcium 30g	•	Iron 0%
Vitamin D 25g		

*Percent Daily Values are based on a 2,000 calorie diet. Your daily values may be higher or lower depending on your calorie needs:

	Calories	2,000	2,500
Total Fat	Less than	65g	80g
Sat Fat	Less than	20g	25g
Cholesterol	Less than	300mg	300mg
Sodium	Less than	2,400 mg	2,400mg
Total Carbohydrate		300g	375g
Dietary Fiber		25g	30g

Ingredients: Lowfat milk, vitamin A palmitate, vitamin D_3.

fat foods, fat is decreased less than 50%. Skim milk, a third variety of milk, is fat free. The label has five parts. Part one describes the serving size, the number of servings in the container, the caloric value of a serving, and the number of calories from fat. The second part indicates the amount of total and saturated fat, cholesterol, sodium, total carbohydrate, dietary fiber and sugar, and protein in both absolute amounts per serving and as a percentage of daily diet containing 2,000 kcal. The third part lists five nutrients (vitamin A, calcium, vitamin D, vitamin C, iron). The fourth part shows the percentage of daily values in a diet containing 2,000 or 2,500 kcal. The final part of the label, at the bottom, lists ingredients in order of weight.

Now that you know what a nutrition label looks like, use it! For the next week, start reading nutrition labels. Keep samples from the packages you bring home, and see how the caloric values compare with other charts.

Once you get in the habit, the nutrition label can be an important aid in maintaining an 'eye' on your calorie intake. Write down the foods you eat for which nutrition labels are inadequate, and use the calorie counting form to help you.

What did you learn by reading labels?

- Labels list ingredients (in decreasing order by weight). If not on container, this must be furnished upon request.
- Labels also tell you about serving size in various containers.
- Labels stress caloric awareness and varying sugar contents, as in canned fruits. (Dietetic foods are the same as regular food except they are sugarless or are made with sugar substitute.)

Helpful Tools

We have already given you two ways to monitor your energy or calorie intake. However, because different ways work better for some people than for others, there are two other methods. Unless food portions are carefully chosen, they can lead to calorie confusion. For this reason, we encourage you to get samples of a few of the food models in portion sizes and keep them at home. In this way, you can get a feeling of the 'size' of the food you are buying or preparing.

To illustrate this: if you buy two oranges, one 2 inches in diameter and the other 2.2 inches, the number of calories in the larger orange is almost 50% more than the smaller one. Thus, food models help you understand what is meant by a 'portion.'

As a final way of dealing with calories, we encourage you to purchase a small scale for weights up to 1 pound and a measuring cup. With such a scale, you can keep accurate records of calories. These scales are available in most health food stores and many stationery stores.

Carbohydrates

These include the sugars and starches in foods. They are a major source of energy and often are immediately available for 'quick' energy. Excess carbohydrates are stored in the liver and muscle, or may be turned into fat if they are not needed.

Carbohydrates yield 4 calories per gram when undergoing chemical changes in the body. This figure can be used to calculate caloric content from nutrition labels on food packages.

All starches and sugars (but not cellulose or fiber) can be converted by digestive juices into simple sugars, one of which is called 'glucose' or dextrose. Some of the glucose (or blood sugar) is used directly as fuel by the tissues of the brain, nervous system, and muscle. This sugar is essential to proper function of your nervous system.

Some of the glucose is converted to glycogen (the storage form of glucose) by the liver and muscles for a quick ready supply of energy when needed. The amount of glycogen is small: only about 250 g (about 1/2 pound or 8 oz).

You can produce glucose from carbohydrates or proteins, but *not* from fat. In starvation, tissues use fat in place of glucose as a source of energy. Hence, survival can be maintained without carbohydrates.

Any excess calories eaten as carbohydrates are converted to fat and stored throughout the body in fat deposits as reserve energy.

Starches can be ranked by the ease with which they are digested and how quickly the glucose appears in the blood. High-glycemic-index starches are digested and absorbed more rapidly. The higher rise in glucose may provoke more insulin release and possibly more hunger. Some suggest emphasizing low-glycemic-index foods.

Cellulose includes the 'fiber' or the 'roughage' in foods and is generally undigestible, or only partially digestible. The cellulose remaining in your intestine forms part of the waste material that retains water and provides bulk to stools. It aids in healthy bowel movements. Fiber may help reduce bowel disease by preventing waste from remaining in the bowel for many days.

Fiber is contained in the seeds, skins, and pulp of fruits, and in vegetables and grains. 'Refining' and 'processing' of food often destroys cellulose. Hence, raw vegetables, fruits, and whole-grain products are preferable to processed foods as sources of fiber.

Many doctors recommend that 45% to 50% of daily calories be in the form of carbohydrates. You may wish to estimate the percentage of carbohydrates in your diet in the coming weeks. Some weight-reduction programs restrict carbohydrate. We examine this concept in detail later.

Carbohydrate foods are healthiest when they contain the least amount of refined sugars and highly processed starches. This is largely true because, in the natural state, they also contain other nutrients.

Eating large amounts of refined sugars and processed starches may be related to dental caries and to diseases of the large intestine.

Proteins

You need protein from both animal and plant sources. Next to water (60%) and fat (20%+), protein is the third most plentiful substance in the body (about 20%). Proteins are major components of body cells. Proteins are essential for repair and replacement of muscles, blood, skin, hair, nails, brain, and other nervous system cells. They can be used as a source of heat and energy, yielding 4 calories a gram. Thus, proteins have the same energy value as carbohydrates. However, if fat and carbohydrate are available in the diet, protein is 'spared,' that is, protein will not be broken down as rapidly by the body to make carbohydrates or fat. Excess protein, however, is converted into fat and stored as body fat.

The digestive process breaks down proteins into amino acids. Approximately 20 amino acids are needed by the body to make all of its proteins, hormones, and enzymes in its many cells. The body can manufacture all but eight of these amino acids from simpler chemicals. These are called *essential amino acids*, since they must be obtained from food.

Foods containing all eight essential amino acids are called *complete protein* foods. These include most meats, eggs, and dairy products. Some vegetable proteins also are complete proteins. Soy protein is an example.

Proteins that lack some of the essential amino acids (or are very low in them) are called *incomplete protein* foods. The proteins found in most fruits, vegetables, and cereal grains are incomplete. By eating a proper combination of vegetable proteins (corn, wheat, and rice), particularly if some proteins from beans (soybeans) are eaten, all the essential amino acids can be obtained.

Protein-containing foods, especially meat, are expensive. The body needs milk (for protein and calcium), which is why dairy products and meats (or high-protein vegetables such as lima, soy, and red beans) are given status as a separate food group.

- Doctors recommend at least 45 to 56 g of protein a day, and more for growing children and pregnant or lactating women. This amounts to about 12% of our calories. Most Americans, and in particular men, eat nearly twice this much protein.
- Because of their high cholesterol content, eggs should be limited to no more than 2 or 3 a week, particularly in men.
- Certain vegetables and seeds of plants, such as legumes and nuts, have high-quality protein. Soy beans and other beans deserve special mention. Vegetable proteins cost much less than meat protein.
- Eggs, cheese, and milk are included in your diet. You can get adequate protein from *carefully chosen* vegetarian diets.

Fats

Fats (also called lipids) are available from both plant and animal sources. They are the most concentrated source of energy. They dissolve other fatty substances, and thus carry the fat-soluble vitamins A, D, E, and K.

Fatty tissues are needed to cushion the internal organs. Fats also aid in insulating the body for better heat maintenance.

Most edible fats are composed of triglycerides, and triglycerides are mainly composed of fatty acids. There are three different types of fatty acids.

Saturated Fatty Acids

These fatty acids often are the chief component of animal fats, including meats and dairy products. They generally do not melt at room temperature. They may raise cholesterol levels in blood. Not all saturated fats are solids, however. Fats such as coconut oil and palm kernel oil are saturated and yet, because of their chemistry, are liquids.

Monounsaturated Fatty Acids

Monounsaturated fatty acids are most common in plant oils. They neither raise nor lower blood cholesterol—olive oil and canola oil are particularly good sources.

Polyunsaturated Fatty Acids

These fatty acids are found in the oils from most common plants, such as corn, soybean, cottonseed, and safflower oils. They are liquid at room temperature and help lower blood cholesterol levels.

Hydrogenated Fats and Trans Fatty Acids

Trans fatty acids are chemical variants of normal (cis) fatty acids. They occur naturally, but mainly result from hydrogenation of polyunsaturated fats that make them solid at room temperature. Trans fatty acids increase the risk of heart disease.

Hydrogenated fats are unsaturated fats with hydrogen chemically added to them. This is done to make them solid and to increase the shelf life (decrease spoilage). Hydrogenated fats also may raise blood cholesterol.

Cholesterol

Cholesterol is another component of animal and plant fats. It can be manufactured in the body, and can also come from the diet, especially the yolks of eggs and the higher-fat, red meats.

One form of cholesterol in the blood, LDL cholesterol or 'bad' cholesterol, is related to the development of heart attacks resulting from hardening of the arteries. In this condition (atherosclerosis), patches of material containing cholesterol form on the inside lining of blood vessels, producing narrowing of the arteries. This increases workload on the heart and increases the risk that patches may close off or block a small artery, producing a heart attack or stroke. A second form of cholesterol in the blood,

HDL cholesterol or 'good' cholesterol, may help prevent heart attacks.

Elevated cholesterol levels (over 200) can be reduced by decreasing the intake of saturated fats (meats and animal protein) and by increasing the intake of monounsaturated and polyunsaturated fats in diets, and by replacing fats with more fruits and vegetables.

Losing weight lowers elevated triglyceride levels.

Five percent to 7% of total calories each day should be from polyunsaturated fat.

Water

Water is the most plentiful component in the body. In both normal and overweight individuals, water represents 60% to 75% of the total weight of the human body.

Each day water is lost in the urine, through the skin as sweat, and in the air. In turn, the body gets its water from drinks, from the water that is part of many foods, and from the water made during chemical changes to food in the body.

For example, each pound of burned fat produces slightly more than a pound of water. Until this water is excreted, weight gain can actually occur while burning fat.

Drinking water during meals provides an important part of the daily need for water, and can provide a break between bites of food. We encourage you to drink at least 8 ounces of water with each meal. This may need to be increased in hot weather or during exercise.

Food Pyramid and Nutrition

One of the simplest approaches to evaluating food intake is the Food Pyramid. During World War II, to make nutrition easier for consumers, foods in supermarkets were divided into seven food groups. In the postwar period, this concept of grouping food was simplified to the Food Group System. This was in turn recently formulated into a pyramid, with the breads, cereals, grains,

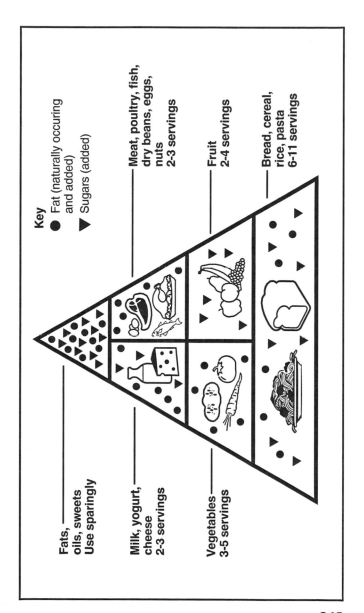

Key
● Fat (naturally occuring and added)
▼ Sugars (added)

Fats, oils, sweets
Use sparingly

Milk, yogurt, cheese
2-3 servings

Vegetables
3-5 servings

Meat, poultry, fish, dry beans, eggs, nuts
2-3 servings

Fruit
2-4 servings

Bread, cereal, rice, pasta
6-11 servings

Table of Food Groups

Food Group	Recommended Daily Servings	Examples
Bread, cereal, rice, and pasta	6-11	Bread Bun (hamburger or hot dog) English muffin Dinner roll Pancake Cooked cereal, rice noodles
Vegetables and fruits	3-5 2-4	Cooked or canned vegetables Cooked or canned fruits (water-packed) Raw orange, apple, banana, or potato Grapefruit Cantaloupe Raw salad greens
Milk, yogurt, and cheese	2-3 (adult)	Whole milk Low-fat (2%) milk Skim milk Ice milk Yogurt, plain w/o fruit Cheese Cottage cheese, creamed Ice cream
Meat, poultry, fish, dry beans, eggs, and nuts	2-3	Cooked lean meat, poultry or fish Hot dogs Luncheon meats Tuna fish (oil pack) (water pack) Eggs Dried beans or peas Nuts Peanut butter

Serving Size	Kilocalories per Serving	Main Contribution to Health
1 slice	60	
1/2 bun	56	B vitamins
1/2 muffin	70	Fiber
1 roll	60-120	
1 (4-inch)	70-105	
1/2 cup	65-100	
1/2 cup	25-100	
1/2 cup	30-100	Vitamins
1 medium	70-95	Minerals
1/2 medium	40	
1/4 medium	30	Fiber
1 cup	20	
1 cup (8 oz)	160	
1 cup	140	Calcium
1 cup	90	
2/3 cup	135-140	
1 cup	120-150	Protein
1-1/3 oz	80-120	
2 oz	60	
1 1/3 cups	340-500	
2 oz	50-125	
2	250	
2 oz	120-190	
2 oz	120	Protein
2 oz	75	
2	160	
1 cup (cooked)	160-230	
1/2 cup	400-600	
4 T	345	

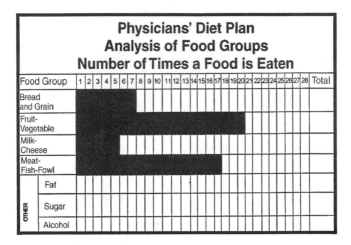

Physicians' Diet Plan
Analysis of Food Groups
Number of Times a Food is Eaten

Food Group	1	2	3	4	5	6	7	8	9	10	11	12	13	14	15	16	17	18	19	20	21	22	23	24	25	26	27	28	Total
Bread and Grain																													
Fruit-Vegetable																													
Milk-Cheese																													
Meat-Fish-Fowl																													
OTHER Fat																													
OTHER Sugar																													
OTHER Alcohol																													

and pasta at the bottom. Fruits and vegetables are next; meats, chicken, poultry, nuts, milk, and cheese are on the third layer, and miscellaneous items are at the top.

These food groups provide a basic guide to good nutrition. The accompanying table shows the food groups with serving sizes and their nutrients.

Physicians' Diet Plan: Monitor for Calories

Day: _____

Food Eaten	Bread, Grains, Cereal, and Rice	Fruits and Vegetables	Milk and Cheese	Meat and Fish	Other

For adults, five servings a day of fruits and vegetables are recommended. Their main nutritional contribution is vitamins, minerals, and, in some cases, fiber. Note the considerable discrepancy between caloric values in this category, although it is not as great as in the milk or meat groups. For example, one serving from raw greens or cantaloupe contains 20 or 30 calories, while servings of an apple, banana, or potato can be 80 calories.

Six to 11 servings of breads, cereals, grains, and pastas are desirable for optimal nutrition. In this group the spread of calories is small, ranging from 60 to 120 calories a serving.

The same nutritional value can be obtained from 8 ounces of milk as from 2 cups of ice cream, yet 2 cups of skim milk contain 90 calories and the corresponding nutritional unit for ice cream has 380 calories.

Physicians' Diet Plan: Monitor for High/Low Food Groups

Day: _____

Food Eaten	Food Group	High	Low

Table of Food Groups in Relation to Calories

Food Group Servings	Relative Calorie (Energy) Value	
	Low	
Bread, cereal, rice, pasta (6-11 servings)	Bread	
	Melba toast	
	Dry nonsugared cereals	
	Cooked grain cereals	
Vegetables and fruits (2-5 servings)	Asparagus	Apple juice
	Beets	Apricots
	Broccoli	Cantaloupe
	Cabbage	Berries
	Celery	Boysenberries
	Chard-spinach	Cranberries
	Cucumber	Lemon
	Green beans	Gooseberries
	Greens	Grapefruit
	Lettuce	Oranges
	Mushrooms	Papayas
	Pickles (dill or sour)	Peaches
	Summer squash	Strawberries
	Tomatoes	Watermelon
	Turnips	
	Winter squash	

The meat, poultry, fish, and beans group includes meat, fish, eggs, dried nuts, and peas. Low-calorie items in this group have less than 50 calories/ounce. The high-calorie foods for an appropriate serving, on the other hand, can range as high as 400 or 500 calories with nuts or peanut butter.

The miscellaneous group (not included in table) contains fats, sugar, and alcohol, with little else in the way of nutrition. These differences among energy values of

High

Biscuits, muffins, rolls
Cornbread and grits
Crackers
Cookies, pie
Pasta (macaroni, noodles, etc)
Tortillas
Doughnuts

Lima beans	Apple	50 kcal/100 g raw
Peas	Banana	vegetable or fruit
Potatoes	Cherries	
Sweet potatoes	Grape juice	
	Grapes	
	Guava	
	Mango	
	Pears	
	Pineapple	
	Plums	
	Prunes	
	Raspberries	

(continued on next page)

foods providing the same overall nutritional values is largely attributable to differences in fat content. This group includes butter, margarine, cooking oil, mayonnaise, and foods like potato chips that have fat but little or no other nutritional value. Also included are sugar-sweetened beverages, sweetened gelatin, candies, pastries, and cakes. Wine, beer, and other alcoholic beverages also are part of this group.

Table of Food Groups in Relation to Calories
(continued)

Food Group Servings	Relative Calorie (Energy) Value	
	Low	
Milk, yogurt, cheese (2 servings for adults, 3 servings for children)	Skim milk Lowfat milk Buttermilk Yogurt (skim milk, without fruit)	
Meat, fish, poultry, and dry beans (2-3 servings)	Liver Chicken Shellfish (shrimp, crab, clams, oyster, lobster)	Abalone Bass Cod Flounder Pike Halibut (California) Swordfish Tuna (water pack) Haddock Perch Trout (brook)

Food Groups

For the next week, identify the food group for the foods you eat using the sample shown above. The tool is the same monitor design you have used before. On the left is a place to write down the foods you eat. On the right are five columns, one for each of the four food groups, and one for the miscellaneous group. Every time you eat, immediately write down what food groups the foods on your plate come from. To help keep track of the days in the week, a small box appears in the top left-hand corner. At the end of the week we will examine your nutrition by food groups.

High

Cottage cheese		60 kcal/100 g
Whole milk		
Ice cream		
Evaporated milk		
Goat milk		
Cheese		
Beef	Herring	150 kcal/100 g raw
Ham	(Atlantic)	
Lamb	Sardines	
Pork	Trout	
Bologna	(rainbow)	
Hot dogs	Tuna (oil	
Turkey	pack)	
Veal	Salmon	
Egg	Whitefish	

A Week Passes

Analyzing Your Food Groups

Now that you have completed a week of recording the foods you have eaten, you can analyze them. The procedure is similar to the ones used before. The recording form is shown above. For each day, check a box for each time you ate a serving of food from that food group. Record the miscellaneous group under the headings of fat, sugar, and alcohol by checking the boxes.

With this information, you can tell which groups did best and which did worst. Equally important, you can get an idea of the number of times you ate something that you recorded in the miscellaneous or 'other' group. You are now ready to begin to control the foods in the latter group.

High-Low Calorie Food Groups: A Modification of the Food Group System

Let us now examine the relationship between nutrition and calories. The High-Low Calorie Food Chart helps you do this. It can be used in shopping and to help control calories and select foods for good nutrition. It is a way to select low-calorie foods within each nutritional group.

The above chart shows the High-Low Calorie Food Guide with the food groups and high-low subdivisions.

At the top of this list are the food groups. The lower part of the sheet contains the breakdown of foods by high and low caloric value. As an approach to shopping and to selecting foods, many foods are divided into high- and low-calorie categories, as well as into food groupings. These are shown in the next table.

In the fruits and vegetables group, the lower-calorie items are generally berries, cantaloupe, tomatoes, and the chewy vegetables. The high-calorie fruits and vegetables tend to include those that are soft and easy to chew, such as bananas, cherries, dried fruits, watermelons, sweet potatoes, etc.

In the bread group, simple pieces of bread, toast, and crackers are in the low-calorie group, while those made with higher fat content—pastries, pies, rolls, muffins, and biscuits—are included in the high-calorie group.

In the milk group, low-calorie foods have had their butterfat content removed.

In the meat group, low-calorie foods are fish, poultry, liver, and veal. High-calorie meats include most of the red meats, frankfurters, eggs, and the redder fishes.

The miscellaneous or 'other' group contains fats, sugars, and alcohol. No low-calorie group exists because these are strictly sugar- or fat-containing groups based on the quantity.

The grouping was done as follows:

Group 1: Breads, cereals, rice, and pasta: the low-calorie designation has 75 calories or less a serving. The high-calorie serving has more than 75 calories.

Group 2: Fruits and vegetables are divided using the half-cup measure. The low-calorie foods have less than 50 calories/half cup, and high-calorie foods have more than 50 calories/half cup.

Group 3: Milk, yogurt, and cheese group: low-calorie items are those with less than 100 calories a serving. The high-calorie foods have more than 100 calories a serving (8 oz).

Group 4: Meat, fish, poultry, dry bean, and egg group: the low-calorie items have less than 50 calories/oz and some (shellfish) have 50 calories/2 oz. The high-calorie items contain 75 calories/oz or more except for luncheon meats, duck, goose, and sweetbreads.

Physicians' Diet Plan
Analysis of High and Low Food Groups
Number of Times a Food is Eaten

Food Group		1	2	3	4	5	6	7	8	9	10	11	12	13	14	15	16	17	18	19	20	21	22	23	24	25	26	27	28	Total
Bread and Grain	Hi																													
	Low																													
Fruit-Vegetable	Hi																													
	Low																													
Milk-Cheese	Hi																													
	Low																													
Meat-Fish-Fowl	Hi																													
	Low																													
MISCELLANEOUS	Fat																													
	Sugar																													
	Alcohol																													

Miscellaneous-Other
Group: Fat, sugar, alcohol: The fat foods include
butter, margarine, cooking oil, mayonnaise,
and potato chips. This group also contains
foods that are predominantly sugar, eg,
sugar-sweetened beverages, candies, pastries, and cakes. Finally, all alcoholic beverages are in this group. Foods are not sepa-
rated by caloric content.

Below is a form you can use for recording food groups
and the high-low calorie nutrients you eat for the next week.

A Week Passes

Keep a list of the foods you eat on the monitor like the
one shown here. Divide them by food groups as outlined
above, and whether they are from the high or low part of
the chart. Analyze the 7 days of records on the form below,
which gives you a way to record the number of high-calorie and low-calorie foods from each group you ate on each
day. A sample is shown below. After seeing the breakdown,
you can decide how you can change the types of foods you
buy or eat to increase the number of low-calorie foods.

Physicians' Diet Plan
Analysis of High and Low Food Groups
Number of Times a Food is Eaten

Food Group		1	2	3	4	5	6	7	8	9	10	11	12	13	14	15	16	17	18	19	20	21	22	23	24	25	26	27	28	Total
Bread and Grain	Hi																													
	Low																													
Fruit-Vegetable	Hi																													
	Low																													
Milk-Cheese	Hi																													
	Low																													
Meat-Fish-Fowl	Hi																													
	Low																													
MISCELLANEOUS	Fat																													
	Sugar																													
	Alcohol																													

Appendix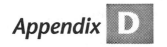

Energy and Exercise

Energy is the ability to do work. The energy your body needs comes from food. Your body uses only what it needs to do its daily work. This includes basal metabolism, which approximates two thirds of your total energy needs: used in digesting food, making and destroying cells, removing waste, breathing, circulating the blood, and maintaining temperature. Any extra energy above what is needed is stored as fat.

On the other hand, if you take less food energy than you need, the body calls on the energy stored in fat. In this way you lose weight. This idea of a balance between

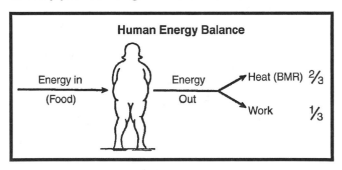

Human Energy Balance

Energy in (Food)

Energy Out

Heat (BMR) ⅔

Work ⅓

what you eat and what you need, with your fat stores serving as a buffer, is depicted below.

Basal metabolism is affected by various factors. It decreases with age. Males have a higher basal metabolism than females. Hormones, such as thyroid hormones, can influence basal metabolism. A cold environment can increase it.

Work, which includes activities such as moving, talking, chewing, and running, is variable and uses approximately one third of the total energy each day. This energy use is directly related to body weight and increases with rate of exercise.

Any fuel as a food that is eaten and not used for metabolism or work is *stored* as *fat*. Approximately 12% to 18% of body weight for men and 25% to 35% for women is fat. It serves as insulation, cushioning, and for emergency needs.

When *less* fuel is taken in than what the body uses, the internal or stored energy is consumed. During starvation, tissues are broken down and used for fuel.

Energy *needs* are *continuous*, but energy *intake* is *sporadic*. Thus, energy constantly shifts into and out of storage depots (ie, a dynamic state).

Increasing Activity

Begin by reviewing your energy needs. This is done by referring to the Energy Balance Diagram.

As we indicated earlier, the only source of energy for the body is from food, and that energy value of food is measured in calories. All the food you eat is digested, and the energy it contains is processed within the body for daily needs.

The law of energy intake and output shows that when you steadily eat more calories than your body needs each day, you store body fat.

Two routes are important for using up energy: body *metabolism* and *daily activity*.

Your body's *basal* or *resting metabolism* accounts for about two thirds of total daily energy expenditure. The beating of your heart and the chemical changes that occur in your kidneys, brain, intestines, etc. are major contributors to resting metabolic needs. If your basal metabolism rate slows down (and it does at every decade of your life), and you fail to convert to energy the calories you consume, they will be stored as fat.

Daily activity accounts for the other significant share of energy used. This usually constitutes about one third of total energy needs.

The quantity of energy used by your body for activity goes up as body weight increases. Thus, overweight people do more work when they walk about a room, get out of a chair, or get dressed than does a person of the same height, sex, and age of normal weight. As a consequence, overweight people tend to perspire more readily, and frequently find activity unpleasant, if not downright uncomfortable.

The energy required for activity increases with the duration, intensity, and rate of activity as well.

There are two ways to look at activity:
1. Activity can be related to calories in food.

Table 7 in Chapter 8 shows the caloric equivalent of several foods, as well as the number of minutes of walking required to burn up extra calories. Note that the heavier you are, the fewer minutes you must walk to burn a given amount of food. Because of the extra weight, however, the insulating effect makes you feel warmer, often discouraging the effort.
2. Activity can be related to *various levels* of activity as well as to the type of activity.

Levels of Activity

Score

0 Sleeping

1 Reclining watching television, reading quietly

2 Very light seated or standing occupations such as painters, cab and truck drivers, laboratory workers, typists, musicians, stitchers, office workers

     Men Office workers, most professional occupations

Women	Office workers, housewives with mechanical aids (eg, dishwashers), teachers, and most other professional women
3 Light	Walking on level at 2.5-3 mph, tailors, pressers, garage work, electricians, carpentry, restaurant trades, cannery workers, manual clothes washing, shopping with light load, golf, sailing, table tennis, volleyball
Men	Most men in light industry, students, building workers except for heavy laborers, many farmers
Women	Light industry, housewives without mechanical appliances, department-store workers, students
4 Moderate	Walking 3.5-4 mph, plasterers, weeding and hoeing, scrubbing floors, loading and stacking heavy loads, shopping with a heavy load, bicycling, skiing, tennis, dancing
Men	Some agricultural workers, unskilled laborers, forestry workers (except lumberjacks), soldiers, miners, steelworkers
Women	Some farm workers, dancers, athletes
5 Heavy	Walking uphill with a load, lumberjack, pick-and-shovel work, basketball, swimming, climbing, football
Men	Lumberjacks, blacksmiths, rickshaw-pullers
Women	Construction workers

This table, from the Recommended Dietary Allowance of the National Academy of Sciences, shows the energy levels related to various activities. From sleeping to the highest levels of activity, the energy expenditure may go up as much as 10 times. However, note also that almost no time is spent in high-level activities, but that nearly 75% of the day is spent on activities with very low levels of energy expenditure.

The Activity Monitor

For the next week, learn more about how much energy you use each day in activity. Record your activity each day for the next week with the Activity Monitor shown below.

Physicians' Diet Plan: Activity Monitor					
Day: ___					
Hour	Activity Level	Hour	Activity Level	Hour	Activity Level
12-1 a.m.		8-9		4-5	
1-2		9-10		5-6	
2-3		10-11		6-7	
3-4		11-12		7-8	
4-5		12-1 p.m.		8-9	
5-6		1-2		9-10	
6-7		2-3		10-11	
7-8		3-4		11-12	

For each day of the week, record the number (0-5) of the activity level during each hour. Use the table above for a detailed listing of the scores and activity.

At the end of each hour (upon arising, for the hours spent sleeping) record the number (0-5) for the highest

Physicians' Diet Plan: Analysis for Activity

Level	Day							Aver-age	Calories per Hour	Level	
	1	2	3	4	5	6	7				
0 Sleeping									——	Basal	
1 Reclining										1	
2 Very Light										2	
3 Light										3	
4 Moderate										4	
5 Heavy										5	
										Total	

Physicians' Diet Plan: Analysis for Activity

Level	Day							Aver-age	Calories per Hour	Level	
	1	2	3	4	5	6	7				
0 Sleeping	8	9	6	7	9	8	9	8	—	Basal	0
1 Reclining	5	3	7	4	6	6	4	5	46	1	230
2 Very Light	8	10	9	10	11	7	8	9	54	2	648
3 Light	2	3	1	2	1	1	4	2	72	3	144
4 Moderate	1	0	2	1	1	0	2	1	100	4	100
5 Heavy	0	0	0	0	0	0	0	0	154	5	0
										Total	1,122

level of activity engaged in for at least 15 minutes of that hour. The numbers in the table provide the basis for the scoring.

Next week, you will use these numbers to calculate how much energy you use in normal activities.

A Week Passes

Analyzing Your Activity

Now that you have finished a week of recording of your activity on an hour-by-hour basis, let's see how many calories you need to account for this activity. Note that the word 'activity' is included both for the muscular activities of which you are aware, and for the resting metabolic activity or energy expended while you are resting or actually asleep.

To analyze the activity you recorded for the past week, we will use the forms above, as well as the two tables that follow, for analysis.

For the first day, add the number of hours spent at each of the five levels of activity, and put these totals under day 1 of the chart. The total hours for that day and for other days should obviously add up to 24. Repeat for the rest of the days until you have determined the number of hours spent for the week at each level. Then average the totals for each day to come up with an average daily total at each level.

Now turn to the table for basal energy. This table relates your height, weight, and age to the average energy expenditure for basal calories.

Basal Energy Needs For Men

Height (in)	Weight (lb)	Age		
		18-35	36-55	56-75
60-65	160	1240	1171	1093
	200	1550	1464	1367
	240	1860	1757	1640
66-71	180	1492	1376	1286
	220	1824	1682	1572
	260	2155	1988	1858
72-78	200	1750	1658	1550
	240	2100	1990	1860
	280	2450	2322	2170

Basal Energy Needs For Women

Height (in)	Weight (lb)	Age		
		18-35	36-55	56-75
60-65	120	900	821	772
	160	1200	1094	1030
	200	1500	1367	1288
	240	1800	1640	1545
66-71	140	1108	1000	945
	180	1388	1286	1215
	220	1668	1572	1485
	260	1972	1858	1755
72-78	160	1380	1240	1166
	200	1600	1550	1458
	240	1910	1860	1750
	280	2240	2170	2042

First, find your age group, and circle all the numbers in that column. Then find your height group and circle the entire row of numbers. Your two circles should locate one group of numbers. Finally, find the weight closest to your own in the column adjacent to your height. Draw a line under all of the numbers that line up in a row with your weight-height group. In the circle made by your age group, this line identifies the basal metabolism nearest to your own. When you arrive at the value for your basal metabolism, record that number on the right-hand side on the Analysis of Activity form.

How to Estimate Calories Spent Through Various Activities

In contrast to the earlier table, the following table is *not* divided according to sex or height. The only variable is weight.

Energy Expenditure in Relation to Body Weight and Activity Level

Activity Level	Weight (lb)			
	120	160	200	240
	Calories per hour			
1	28	37	46	55
2	32	43	54	65
3	43	58	72	86
4	60	80	100	120
5	92	123	154	184

If you weigh 180 pounds, the values are between those under columns for 160 and 200 pounds. Thus, at activity level 1, you spend approximately 41 calories/hour, at level 2 approximately 47, at level 3, 65, at level 4, 90, and at level 5, 138. However, these are estimates. The numbers are now transferred to the column labeled calories per hour, which is adjacent to the column labeled average. Multiply the average number of hours at each level by the calories/hour for this level, and write the number on the column at the far right. A sample is shown above. The number in the grand total should give a reasonable estimate of the number of calories you expended during the past week. Since you recorded an activity level with only 15 minutes of time spent at that level, this first grand total is obviously an overestimate. If you want to be more accurate, repeat the same recording monitor and record the level when you spend 45 minutes or more at a given level. This additional information, which should be lower than the previous one, yields a good estimate for the range of energy you need to maintain your body.

A Word About Exercise

Although increased activity may be good for you, any sudden change, particularly if you have been inactive in the past months or years, can cause trouble. Before increasing your activity level by introducing activities you are not already doing, you are strongly advised to consult with your physician to obtain clearance to engage in new or more strenuous levels of physical activity.

You can perform at least two kinds of exercises. The first is aerobic, and the second is anaerobic.

Aerobic exercises involve such things as walking, swimming, bicycling, jogging, etc. Anaerobic exercises, on the other hand, tend to involve isometric or muscle-building exercises.

For most people, aerobic exercises are preferred because they increase your metabolism to help burn energy. For overweight people who are able, swimming and bicycling are good activities because your weight is supported by the water or the bicycle seat.

To give you some feeling about the calorie expenditure with various activities, the next table shows the calories used per minute above basal level for different activities. Note that, for many activities, you expend few calories above basal levels. However, if you do any of these activities for a long time, the effect can be important.

We know that activity and movement can be helpful in any weight-control program. For many overweight people walking is most desirable, since it can be done anywhere at almost any time of year, and is a form of activity that we all do. Walking is particularly helpful in maintaining weight loss once it has been achieved. While exercise alone is unlikely to bring about a significant loss of weight, it can help enormously when combined with careful control of food intake.

Energy Expenditure Above Basal Levels Related to Body Weight and Activity

| | Body Weight (lb) | | |
	120	160	200
		Cal/min	
Lying	0.10	0.12	0.15
Sitting	0.38	0.50	0.62
Standing	0.45	0.61	0.77
Ironing	0.90	1.22	1.54
Walking (3 mph)	1.80	2.41	3.03
Carpentry	2.10	2.80	3.50
Bicycling	2.30	3.05	3.80
Calisthenics	2.50	3.35	4.20
Dancing	2.70	3.65	4.60
Walking (4 mph)	3.12	4.12	5.13
Skating	3.20	4.26	5.33
Swimming (2 mph)	7.10	10.05	12.00
Running (10 mph)	12.83	17.06	21.28

The values in this table represent the increase over basal energy expenditure associated with each activity. When you calculated your basal energy earlier, you saw that it changes with age, weight, and height. The values in this table are corrected by subtracting the energy you would spend at basal level from the total associated with each activity. For most people, basal energy is just below 1 calorie/minute. Lying adds little to the extra energy, but standing can increase it by nearly 50% above basal, depending on weight. Your motto should be 'keep moving, no matter how slowly.'

For example, if you increase your activity by as much as 10% to 15% through walking or other activity, your calorie needs can move you up from the classification of sedentary. Moreover, if your exercise program is followed faithfully, you will be able to afford more calories, thus more food, each day without regaining weight.

Even a small amount of walking or other activity each day can make a difference in caloric expenditure. Projecting this over a year, a significant weight loss is involved. On the other hand, if you reduce your activity, you will gain weight unless you also reduce your food.

Exercise implies a number of things. It is the way you move and the way you breathe, as well as the way you walk. It is not something to be done just when you feel like it. Ideally, walking or other activity should be regular and consistent, according to age and gender.

Warming Up
A significant factor in regard to activity is 'warming up.' The following are good examples of simple warm-ups:
1. Relax your arms, let your hands hang limp, then shake your hands.
2. Rotate your arms, leading with the elbows.
3. Rotate your head, permitting the jaw to hang slack. Close your eyes while doing this exercise.
4. Rotate just the shoulders, first together and then separately.

Getting Into Shape
To become more active, your body may need conditioning. Getting into shape is necessary first.

Exercises not only get you into shape, but also keep you supple and limber, improve your muscle tone, relax you, may help correct your posture, and, above all, reduce weight.

Think of your body as a machine. To keep a machine in good working order, you would not permit it to sit idle constantly, would you? In the same way, your body functions better when it is kept in good working order. And your body—because of nature's wonderful powers—will respond positively and become stronger when used properly. If you plan to increase your walking, do it gradually.

Three Keys to Exercise

Before you begin exercising, consider the three things you always do, whether exercising or not: *thinking*, *breathing*, and *posturing*. Make sure that you do them correctly and that you have your doctor's approval before beginning any significant departure from your usual habits of activity.

Thinking Positively

Walking should become a way of life. When you embark on this program, it should be important to want to not only feel better now, but also continue feeling better. Form a mental picture of what you would like to look like and how you would like to feel. Place it alongside the image of what you look like now and how you feel now. This should help motivate you every day.

Breathing Effectively

People use only one eighth of their total lung capacity when breathing normally. Poor breathing habits can further decrease your capacity to walk or do anything else. Adopting good breathing habits is wise because you will find walking or other activities much easier if you breathe properly.

When you breathe, you take oxygen into your lungs and you exhale carbon dioxide. A normal person takes about 16 to 20 breaths a minute, or 23,000 times a day. Our breathing tends to become more 'shallow' the older and heavier we get. Breathing is, of course, vital to your entire body. The more efficiently you breathe, the more efficiently your body functions. There are two methods of deep breathing: (1) breathing through your mouth, drawing air in gasps, and (2) closing your mouth and breathing deeply through your nose. With either method, stand 'large,' spreading your ribs to the side.

Here are some exercises to increase your lung capacity, strengthen your diaphragm, and help you develop good breathing habits:

- Take a deep breath, fill your lungs full, and see how long you can hold that breath. Then, with teeth closed, expel it with a hissing noise. Do this as slowly as possible and finish with one last, forceful hiss. This will help clear your lungs. Repeat this exercise several times or whenever you think of it.
- Take a deep breath and enjoy it. Count to 20 as you exhale. As singers and swimmers know, the amount of air you can hold in your lungs is extremely important.
- Light a candle and hold it about 10 inches from your mouth. Take a deep breath and fill your lungs. Expire the air slowly in such a way as to keep the candle burning. It will waver, but should not be blown out.

Posturing Correctly

To breathe properly, you must sit and stand straight. Obviously, you cannot fill your lungs if they are distorted by your posture. Picture your lungs as two balloons you must fill, one on either side of your chest.

Whether you are sitting or standing, your back should be upright, shoulders back but relaxed, chest and head up. One of the easiest ways of picturing this position is to imagine a string tied to the top of your head and to your chest, puppet fashion. When the string is pulled taut, everything falls into place without much effort.

This position can also be practiced by backing up to a wall. Make an effort to touch the small of your back, your calves, and the back of your heel (in chin-down position) to the wall. Stay in this position and try the deep-breathing exercises. The very few minutes spent on them can benefit you tremendously. In addition, these breathing exercises are necessary for forming a firm foundation for your exercise program, and can be sandwiched into your day easily and frequently.

Begin Slowly

Now you are ready to begin moving your entire body. The important thing to remember is that it is far better to *begin slowly* than to start off with a bang and then not be able to keep it up. Even a limited program can help you feel much better.

Some of you may do no more than what has already been mentioned: the basic warm-ups, breathing, and posturing, and all with a good mental attitude.

You should also *respect your fatigue point.* If, when walking, you feel pain in any part of your body, stop immediately. Never push yourself to continue under these circumstances. Consult with your physician. Your fatigue point is not stationary, however, and you can usually gradually increase the amount of walking.

Nothing is magical about any program for activity. Yours should include some form of aerobic activity. Walking is the most suitable exercise. Learn to think in terms of energy exchange and you need never be overweight again.

Physicians' Diet Plan: Monitor of Activity		
Day: ____		
Activity	Time	
	Start	Stop

To emphasize the importance of energy expenditure in everyday life, we want you to maintain a regular record of the activity you do every day. Using a monitor like the one below, record each time you do activities outside your regular job. The more you move, the more energy (calories) your body can use without gaining weight. Walking is certainly the easiest for most people, and can be done every day. Other activities you normally engage in also should be noted. Remember that if you have no activity above your daily job requirements, then the day should have a zero for extra energy expenditure. As you become more conscious of your activities, the number of days with zero should fall off as the number of days with extra activity increases.

A recording form to record the number of times you perform various activities is shown below. Record each time you spent more than the listed time at an activity. Remember, to reach and maintain your weight goal, you need to substitute activities such as walking for times you might eat. Eating on the move is harder than when standing still. So keep moving!

Physicians' Diet Plan
Analysis for Activity
Number of Times

	Number of Times													
	1	2	3	4	5	6	7	8	9	10	11	12	Add'l	Total
Walking (30 minutes)														
Down stairs														
Up stairs														
Cycling (15 minutes)														
Swimming (15 minutes)														
Jogging (15 minutes)														

Index

A

acanthosis nigricans 92, 145

Accutrim 253

acrocephaly 117

acromegaly 110

Addison's disease 63

Adipex-P® 251

adiposis dolorosa 106

adiposity rebound 123

adipsin (complement D) 55, 56, 83

adjustable gastric banding 275

adrenal insufficiency 107, 108

aerobics 230

agitation 263

AIDS 112

alcohol 51, 52, 212, 214, 220

Alström syndrome 117

amenorrhea 107-109, 146

amino acids 206, 217, 268

aminorex 150, 247, 262

amitriptyline (Elavil®) 111

amoxapine 111

amphetamine (Dexedrine®) 150, 246, 247, 250, 260

amylin 268

anastomotic leak 282

androgens 82, 84, 269

anemia 282, 284

anger 180

angiotensinogen 55, 56

antiandrogen 270

antiepileptics 111

antipsychotics 110, 111

anxiety 180

aortic regurgitation 266

aortic valvulopathy 264

apomorphine 249

apoptosis 37

arginine 206

arthritis 277

glucocorticoids 40, 41, 63, 111

Glucophage® 112

glucose 51, 56, 59, 86-88, 93, 105, 114, 128, 136, 145-147, 149, 202, 210, 215, 216, 218, 243, 268, 271, 286

glyburide (DiaBeta®, Glynase®, Micronase®) 112

glycemic index 210

glycerol 215

glycogen 54, 115, 202, 217, 220, 231

Glynase® 112

gout 69, 78

growth hormone releasing hormone (GHRH) 58, 61

H

hallucinations 263

haloperidol 111

HDL cholesterol 55, 80, 81, 93, 96, 98, 136, 146, 148, 149, 259

headache 107, 146

heart attack 79, 229

heart disease 11, 28, 69, 77-80, 94, 95, 98, 134, 137, 148, 209, 210, 248, 260, 261, 266

heart failure 73, 92, 97, 146

high-density lipoproteins 243

high-density-lipoprotein (HDL) cholesterol 218, 286

hirsutism 92, 109, 146

histidine 206

house cleaning 239

hydrodensitometry 14, 18

hydrogen 16

hypercholesterolemia 73, 80, 93, 248

hyperglycemia 147

hyperinsulinemia 38, 55, 81, 84, 87, 90, 95

hyperlipidemia 69

hyperphagia 38, 57, 60, 107, 116

M

ma huang 270

Madelung's deformity 106

Maffucci's syndrome 106

magnesium 16, 207

magnetic resonance imaging (MRI) 14, 19, 21, 105, 140

malabsorption 282

malnutrition 282, 284

mania 263

Mazanor® 253

mazindol (Sanorex®, Mazanor®) 249, 252, 255, 256, 259, 266

Medifast 199

megestrol acetate (Megace®) 111, 112

melanin-concentrating hormone (MCH) 58, 61

melanocyte-stimulating hormone (α-MSH) 37-39, 58, 61

menopause 64, 125, 126, 162

mental retardation 116, 119

mepazine 111

Meridia® 160, 253, 255, 256

mesoridazine 111

metabolic syndrome 93, 98, 120, 146

metformin (Glucophage®) 112

methamphetamine (Desoxyn®) 247, 250, 251, 260

methionine 206

Micronase® 112

minerals 13, 16, 17, 206, 211, 220, 284

mismatch model 5

mitral regurgitation 266

monoamine oxidase inhibitors (MAOIs) 259

mood disorders 69

myocardial infarction 92, 160, 271

N

O

Notes

Notes

Notes